T0259626

Cardiac Arrhythmias

Editor

MARY G. CAREY

CRITICAL CARE NURSING CLINICS OF NORTH AMERICA

www.ccnursing.theclinics.com

Consulting Editor
JAN FOSTER

September 2016 • Volume 28 • Number 3

ELSEVIER

1600 John F. Kennedy Boulevard • Suite 1800 • Philadelphia, Pennsylvania, 19103-2899

http://www.theclinics.com

CRITICAL CARE NURSING CLINICS OF NORTH AMERICA Volume 28, Number 3
September 2016 ISSN 0899-5885, ISBN-13: 978-0-323-46254-9

Editor: Kerry Holland
Developmental Editor: Colleen Viola

© **2016 Elsevier Inc. All rights reserved.**

This periodical and the individual contributions contained in it are protected under copyright by Elsevier, and the following terms and conditions apply to their use:

Photocopying
Single photocopies of single articles may be made for personal use as allowed by national copyright laws. Permission of the Publisher and payment of a fee is required for all other photocopying, including multiple or systematic copying, copying for advertising or promotional purposes, resale, and all forms of document delivery. Special rates are available for educational institutions that wish to make photocopies for non-profit educational classroom use. For information on how to seek permission visit www.elsevier.com/permissions or call: (+44) 1865 843830 (UK)/(+1) 215 239 3804 (USA).

Derivative Works
Subscribers may reproduce tables of contents or prepare lists of articles including abstracts for internal circulation within their institutions. Permission of the Publisher is required for resale or distribution outside the institution. Permission of the Publisher is required for all other derivative works, including compilations and translations (please consult www.elsevier.com/permissions).

Electronic Storage or Usage
Permission of the Publisher is required to store or use electronically any material contained in this periodical, including any article or part of an article (please consult www.elsevier.com/permissions). Except as outlined above, no part of this publication may be reproduced, stored in a retrieval system or transmitted in any form or by any means, electronic, mechanical, photocopying, recording or otherwise, without prior written permission of the Publisher.

Notice
No responsibility is assumed by the Publisher for any injury and/or damage to persons or property as a matter of products liability, negligence or otherwise, or from any use or operation of any methods, products, instructions or ideas contained in the material herein. Because of rapid advances in the medical sciences, in particular, independent verification of diagnoses and drug dosages should be made.

Although all advertising material is expected to conform to ethical (medical) standards, inclusion in this publication does not constitute a guarantee or endorsement of the quality or value of such product or of the claims made of it by its manufacturer.

Critical Care Nursing Clinics of North America (ISSN 0899-5885) is published quarterly by Elsevier Inc., 360 Park Avenue South, New York, NY 10010-1710. Months of issue are March, June, September, and December. Business and Editorial Offices: 1600 John F. Kennedy Blvd., Suite 1800, Philadelphia, PA 19103-2899. Periodicals postage paid at New York, NY and additional mailing offices. Subscription prices are $155.00 per year for US individuals, $370.00 per year for US institutions, $100.00 per year for US students and residents, $200.00 per year for Canadian individuals, $464.00 per year for Canadian institutions, $230.00 per year for international individuals, $464.00 per year for international institutions and $115.00 per year for Canadian and international students/residents. To receive student/resident rate, orders must be accompanied by name of affiliated institution, data of term, and the *signature* of program/residency coordinator on institution letterhead. Orders will be billed at individual rate until proof of status is received. Foreign air speed delivery is included in all *Clinics* subscription prices. All prices are subject to change without notice. **POSTMASTER:** Send address changes to *Critical Care Nursing Clinics of North America*, Elsevier Health Sciences Division, Subscription Customer Service, 3251 Riverport Lane, Maryland Heights, MO 63043. **Customer Service: 1-800-654-2452 (US and Canada); 314-447-8871 (outside US and Canada). Fax: 314-447-8029. E-mail:** JournalsCustomerService-usa@elsevier.com **(for print support) and** JournalsOnlineSupport-usa@elsevier.com **(for online support).**

Reprints. For copies of 100 or more of articles in this publication, please contact the Commercial Reprints Department, Elsevier Inc., 360 Park Avenue South, New York, New York, 10010-1710; Tel.: 212-633-3874, Fax: 212-633-3820, and E-mail: reprints@elsevier.com.

Critical Care Nursing Clinics of North America is covered in *MEDLINE/PubMed (Index Medicus), International Nursing Index, Nursing Citation Index, Cumulative Index to Nursing and Allied Health Literature, and RNdex Top 100.*

Contributors

CONSULTING EDITOR

JAN FOSTER, PhD, APRN, CNS
Formerly, Associate Professor, College of Nursing, Texas Woman's University, Houston; President, Nursing Inquiry and Intervention, Inc, The Woodlands, Texas

EDITOR

MARY G. CAREY, PhD, RN, FAHA, FAAN
Associate Director, Clinical Nursing Research Center, Department of Nursing Practice, Strong Memorial Hospital; Associate Professor, University of Rochester School of Nursing, University of Rochester Medical Center, Rochester, New York

AUTHORS

SALAH S. AL-ZAITI, RN, ANP-BC, PhD
Assistant Professor, Department of Acute and Tertiary Care, School of Nursing, University of Pittsburgh, Pittsburgh, Pennsylvania

MINA ATTIN, PhD, RN
Assistant Professor, University of Rochester School of Nursing, Rochester, New York

AKSANA BALDZIZHAR, MD
Project Research Assistant, School of Nursing, University of Rochester Medical Center, Rochester, New York

RAYMOND BOND, PhD
Computing Science Research Institute, School of Computing and Mathematics, University of Ulster, Newtownabbey, County Antrim, Northern Ireland

MARY G. CAREY, PhD, RN, FAHA, FAAN
Associate Director, Clinical Nursing Research Center, Department of Nursing Practice, Strong Memorial Hospital; Associate Professor, University of Rochester School of Nursing, University of Rochester Medical Center, Rochester, New York

DEWAR D. FINLAY, PhD
The Engineering Research Institute (ERI), School of Engineering, University of Ulster at Jordanstown, Newtownabbey, County Antrim, Northern Ireland

J. LEE GARVEY, MD
Director of Emergency Cardiac Care, Carolinas Medical Center, Charlotte, North Carolina

DANIEL GULDENRING, PhD
The Engineering Research Institute (ERI), School of Engineering, University of Ulster at Jordanstown, Newtownabbey, County Antrim, Northern Ireland

PATRICIA R.E. HARRIS, PhD, RN, CNS
Assistant Professor, Department of Nursing, School of Health and Natural Sciences, Dominican University of California, San Rafael, California

ALAN KENNEDY, BSc
The Engineering Research Institute (ERI), School of Engineering, University of Ulster at Jordanstown, Newtownabbey, County Antrim, Northern Ireland

YURY KRYVALAP, MD
Post-doctoral Fellow, Department of Pathology, Strong Memorial Hospital, University of Rochester Medical Center, Rochester, New York

AIMEE LEE, CNS, ACNP-BC
Nurse Practitioner, Cardiac Electrophysiology, Stanford Health Care, Stanford, California

KATHY S. MAGDIC, RN, ACNP-BC, DNP
Assistant Professor, Department of Acute and Tertiary Care, School of Nursing; Coordinator of Adult-Gero ACNP Program, University of Pittsburgh, Pittsburgh, Pennsylvania

EKATERINA MANUYLOVA, MD
Department of Endocrinology, Diabetes and Metabolism, University of Rochester; Assistant Professor, Department of Medicine, Strong Memorial Hospital, University of Rochester Medical Center, Rochester, New York

ROMAN MARCHENKO, MD
Department of Interventional Electrophysiology, Electrophysiologist Interventionalist, Federal Center of Cardiovascular Surgery, Penza, Russia

JAMES McLAUGHLIN, PhD
The Engineering Research Institute (ERI), School of Engineering, University of Ulster at Jordanstown, Newtownabbey, County Antrim, Northern Ireland

SHERRI L. McMULLEN, PhD, FNP, NNP-BC
Assistant Professor, College of Nursing, Upstate Medical University, Syracuse, New York; Research Consultant, Nursing Practice, University of Rochester Medical Center, Rochester, New York

KIERAN MORAN, PhD
School of Health and Human Performance, Dublin City University, Glanevin, Dublin, Ireland

DAVID PICKHAM, RN, PhD, FAHA
Clinical Assistant Professor, General Medical Disciplines, Stanford Medicine, Stanford, California

REBECCA G. TUCKER, PhD, ACNPC, MEd, RN
Clinical Assistant Professor, University of Rochester School of Nursing, Rochester, New York

SHU-FEN WUNG, PhD, RN, ACNP-BC, FAAN
Associate Professor, Biobehavioral Health Science Division, The University of Arizona College of Nursing, Tucson, Arizona

JESSICA K. ZÈGRE-HEMSEY, PhD, RN
Assistant Professor, School of Nursing, University of North Carolina at Chapel Hill, Chapel Hill, North Carolina

Contents

Paroxysmal supraventricular tachycardia (PSVT) is a well-known and thoroughly studied clinical syndrome, characterized by regular tachycardia rhythm with sudden onset and abrupt termination. Most patients present with palpitations and dizziness, and their electrocardiogram demonstrates a narrow QRS complex and regular tachycardia with hidden or inverted P waves. PSVT is caused by re-entry due to the presence of inhomogeneous, accessory, or concealed conducting pathways. Hemodynamically stable patients are treated by vagal maneuvers, intravenous adenosine, diltiazem, or verapamil, hemodynamically unstable patients are treated by cardioversion. Patients with symptomatic and recurrent PSVT can be treated with long-term drug treatment or catheter ablation.

Ventricular tachycardias include ventricular tachycardia, ventricular fibrillation, and torsades de pointes; although these rhythms may be benign and asymptomatic, others may be life threatening and lead to increased morbidity and mortality. To optimize patient outcomes, ventricular tachycardias need to be rapidly diagnosed and managed, and often the electrocardiogram (ECG) is the first and only manifestation of a cardiac defect. Understanding of the initial electrocardiographic pattern and subsequent changes can lead to early intervention and an improved outcome. This article describes mechanisms, ECG characteristics, and management of ventricular tachycardias.

Patients present to the emergency department (ED) with a wide range of complaints, and ED clinicians are responsible for identifying which conditions are life threatening. Cardiac monitoring strategies in the ED include, but are not limited to, 12-lead electrocardiography and bedside cardiac monitoring for arrhythmia and ischemia detection as well as QT-interval monitoring. ED nurses are in a unique position to incorporate cardiac monitoring into the early triage and risk stratification of patients with cardiovascular emergencies to optimize patient management and outcomes.

Acute coronary syndrome (ACS) is caused by a critical obstruction of a coronary artery because of atherosclerotic coronary artery disease. Three specific conditions are included: ST elevation myocardial infarction, non–ST elevation myocardial infarction, and unstable angina. The ST segment on the electrocardiogram is a sensitive and specific marker of myocardial ischemia and infarction; however, ST segment deviation is regional not global, thus the ECG lead must be placed over the affected region of the

CRITICAL CARE NURSING CLINICS OF NORTH AMERICA

FORTHCOMING ISSUES

December 2016
Mechanical Ventilation in the Critically Ill Patient: International Nursing Perspectives
Sandra Goldsworthy, *Editor*

March 2017
Infection in the Intensive Care Unit
Todd Tartavoulle and Jennifer Manning, *Editors*

June 2017
Pediatric Critical Care
Jerithea Tidwell and Brennan Lewis, *Editors*

RECENT ISSUES

June 2016
Sedation and Sleep in Critical Care: An Update
Jan Foster, *Editor*

March 2016
Neuromonitoring and Assessment
Catherine Harris, *Editor*

December 2015
Heart Failure
Jennifer Kitchens and Lenora Maze, *Editors*

ISSUE OF RELATED INTEREST

Cardiac Electrophysiology Clinics
March 2016 (Vol. 8, Issue 2)
Interpretation of Complex Arrhythmias: A Case-Based Approach
Mohammad Shenasa and Stanley Nattel, *Editors*
Available at: http://www.cardiacEP.theclinics.com

THE CLINICS ARE AVAILABLE ONLINE!
Access your subscription at:
www.theclinics.com

Preface
Cardiac Arrhythmias

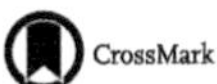

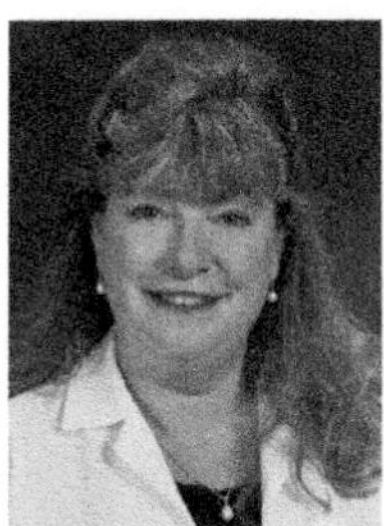

Mary G. Carey, PhD, RN, FAHA, FAAN
Editor

In 1893, Dr Willem Einthoven, from the Netherlands, introduced the word "electrocardiogram" and, over a quarter of a century later, in 1924, was awarded the Nobel Prize for inventing the electrocardiograph. Some ask why ECG rather than EKG. It is because the word electrocardiogram (ECG) in German is spelled elektrokardiographie (EKG). Another common question is, why does the labeling of the waveforms begin with PQRST rather than ABCDE? This convention goes back to Descartes, who used the letter P to denote a point on a curve (for understandable reasons). Einthoven was apparently inspired by this to use PQRST to denote the waves on his early tracings. However, it is not true that PQRST were used from the very beginning; Dr Einthoven apparently also used ABCD to denote waves on early forms of ECG recordings, and, then, as he refined the technique, used PQRST to talk about the new "corrected" recordings. It seems to be a happy coincidence that PQRST left space on either end for the addition of new waves, as they were discovered, like the U wave.

Despite the increasing demands for cardiac imaging, the ECG remains the classic, go-to diagnostic test for cardiac evaluation. As an incredibly valuable tracking tool, ECG recordings are painless and completely noninvasive. When embedded in a wearable or mobile device and accompanied by algorithms, ECG biosensors can shed light on a variety of advanced biometrics, including:

- Heart rate
- Heart rate variability
- Stress
- Fatigue
- Heart age
- Breathing index
- Mood

Crit Care Nurs Clin N Am 28 (2016) ix–x
http://dx.doi.org/10.1016/j.cnc.2016.06.001
0899-5885/16/© 2016 Published by Elsevier Inc.

DEDICATION

To my editor, Dixie Carole Crabtree:

It is upon the scaffold

Of your intellectual acuity,

Your generosity of spirit,

And your endless interest

That this work was completed.

Mary G. Carey, PhD, RN, FAHA, FAAN
Clinical Nursing Research Center
School of Nursing, Strong Memorial Hospital
University of Rochester Medical Center
601 Elmwood Avenue
Box 619-7
Rochester, NY 14642, USA

E-mail address:
Mary_Carey@URMC.Rochester.edu

The Cardiac Conduction System

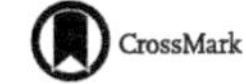

Generation and Conduction of the Cardiac Impulse

Alan Kennedy, BSc[a,*], Dewar D. Finlay, PhD[a], Daniel Guldenring, PhD[a], Raymond Bond, PhD[b], Kieran Moran, PhD[c], James McLaughlin, PhD[a]

KEYWORDS

- Action potential • Cardiac conduction system • Electrocardiogram • Automaticity
- Cardiac impulse

KEY POINTS

- Contraction of the heart is initiated by the generation and conduction of the cardiac impulse.
- Pacemaker cells generate a cardiac impulse without any external stimulation because of changes in electrolyte concentration inside and outside the cell.
- A cardiac impulse is conducted from the sinoatrial node to the atrioventricular node via internodal pathways and passes through the atrioventricular node to depolarize the ventricular myocardium through the Purkinje network.
- Changes in the ionic potential during the heartbeat can be recorded from the surface of the skin, yielding electronic data known as the electrocardiogram.

INTRODUCTION

Cardiac disease is the most common cause of mortality in the developed world, and the number of patient deaths from cardiovascular-related disease increased by a third between 1990 and 2010.[1] This increase, coupled with a further projected increase in the prevalence of cardiovascular disease,[2] has led to the electrocardiogram (ECG)

Disclosure Statement: The authors have nothing to disclose.

[a] The Engineering Research Institute (ERI), School of Engineering, University of Ulster at Jordanstown, Newtownabbey, County Antrim BT37 0QB, Northern Ireland; [b] Computing Science Research Instititute, School of Computing and Mathematics, University of Ulster, Room 16G06, Jordanstown Campus, Shore Road, Newtownabbey BT37 0QB, County Antrim, Northern Ireland; [c] School of Health and Human Performance, Dublin City University, Room XG05, Glanevin, Dublin 9, Ireland

* Corresponding author. University of Ulster, Jordanstown Campus, Shore Road, Newtownabbey BT37 0QB, Co. Antrim, UK.

E-mail addresses: Kennedy-A23@email.ulster.ac.uk; a.kennedy@ulster.ac.uk

Crit Care Nurs Clin N Am 28 (2016) 269–279
http://dx.doi.org/10.1016/j.cnc.2016.04.001 ccnursing.theclinics.com
0899-5885/16/$ – see front matter Crown Copyright © 2016 Published by Elsevier Inc. All rights reserved.

becoming one of the most used tools in clinical practice. To fully understand the ECG and interpret its results, an understanding of the normal conduction system of the heart is necessary.

The human heart contracts approximately 2.5 billion times during the average person's life span; this is accomplished by the cardiac conduction system.[3] The cardiac conduction system is a physiologic system whereby the myocardium (heart muscle) is stimulated to contract without the requirement of any external stimulation. Contraction of a cardiac myocyte (heart cell) is initiated by an electrical impulse (the cardiac impulse), which propagates freely through the atrial and ventricular myocardium. This phenomenon occurs because cardiac myocytes are electrically coupled via, so-called, gap junctions.[4] All of the myocytes within the heart have the capacity to conduct cardiac impulse; this means that a single stimulation of an atrial or ventricular myocyte can produce contraction of the entire myocardium. During normal activation of the heart, the cardiac impulse originates from pacemaker cells within the sinoatrial (SA) node and uniformly spreads through the atria. The cardiac impulse is then conducted to the atrioventricular (AV) node, via internodal pathways, where it spreads throughout the conduction system of the ventricles and the ventricular myocardium. Irregularities in the normal cardiac conduction system can cause cardiac arrhythmias and, therefore, an abnormal ECG. This article outlines the key principles behind a normal cardiac conduction system, including the generation of the cardiac impulse and propagation of this impulse from the atria through a normal conduction system to the ventricular myocardium.

THE UNDERLYING PRINCIPLES BEHIND THE HEARTBEAT

Electrolytes and Concentration Gradients

To understand the cardiac conduction system, it is important to understand the way in which cells, in particular pacemaker and normal cardiac cells, function. The human body is composed of millions of cells, each cell enclosed by a fatty membrane and surrounded by extracellular fluid.[5,6] All components of the cell contain electrolytes. The electrolytic concentration gradient, along with the ability of the electrolytes to cross the cell membrane, allows the generation of an electrical current.[7]

For contraction of a cardiac myocyte, the most important electrolytes are sodium, potassium, and calcium. The electrolytes are moved in and out of the cell through 2 main pathways: (1) pumps embedded in the cell membrane and (2) ion channels in the cell membrane (**Fig. 1**).[8] The sodium potassium pump plays an important role in this process as it moves sodium out of the cell and pumps potassium in. A concentration gradient is created because the pump is continuously pumping potassium into the cell leading to a greater concentration of potassium inside of the cell than outside, resulting in a change in intracellular potential. In this process, the opposite is true for sodium as a greater sodium concentration is created on the outside of the cell with a lesser sodium concentration inside. The other method by which electrolytes move in and out of a cardiac myocyte is through ion channels.[9] Unlike the sodium potassium pump, which allows multiple electrolytes to pass, ion channels are specific to a single electrolyte. Ion channels are voltage gated and allow for each specific electrolyte to move either in or out of the cell depending on the concentration gradient of that particular ion.[10] When potassium channels are opened, potassium leaves the cell; when sodium channels are opened, sodium enters the cell. It is these opposing reactions that result in an electrical charge across the cell membrane. This is, therefore, the underlying principle behind generation of the cardiac impulse.

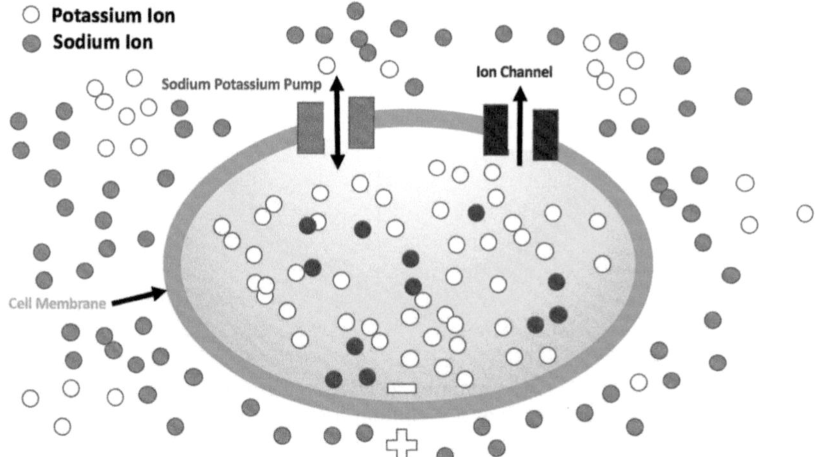

Fig. 1. The ionic components of a cardiac myocyte. The greater concentration of potassium ions inside the cell than outside creates a potential across the cell membrane.

Depolarization and Repolarization

Contraction, and subsequent relaxation of the heart, is achieved through depolarization and repolarization of all the cardiac myocytes. The change in cell membrane permeability directly affects the electrolyte concentration within and surrounding the cell, creating an impulse. This cardiac impulse propagates through surrounding tissues causing depolarization of the entire myocardium. Depolarization involves a surge of electrical current across the cell membrane, which forces a change in the cell's resting potential and generation of an action potential that spreads through the heart. Repolarization is the process by which the cell returns to its normal resting state.

Action Potential of a Cardiac Myocyte

An action potential is a brief change in the voltage across the cell membrane of a muscle or nerve cell when an adequate stimulation is applied. The cardiac action potential is described in 5 main phases (0–4). Phase 4 represents the cell at rest; at this time the cell has a potential of approximately −90 mV.[11] An electrical current from a surrounding myocyte (muscle cell) then stimulates the membrane opening the potassium sodium pump allowing sodium to enter, rapidly altering the potential of the cell from negative (−90 mV) to positive (+20 mV). This phase is known as phase 0 and is, commonly, referred to as the depolarization phase. Next, the calcium channels open allowing calcium to enter the cell creating a slight decrease (phase 1), which is followed by a stabilization in the cell's potential (the plateau phase, phase 2) at approximately +10 mV and closes the sodium channel. Towards the end of phase 2, calcium is released from intracellular stores increasing the concentration of calcium within the cell and causing mechanical contraction. In Phase 3, after contraction, the calcium channels close and potassium channels open causing the cell to repolarize and return to its resting potential of −90 mV.[10] All phases of depolarization and repolarization of a cardiac myocyte can be seen in **Fig. 2**A. Once a cardiac myocyte experiences an action potential, it rapidly spreads from cell to cell. However, once a cell is depolarized it becomes refractory for a short period of time; this, essentially, means

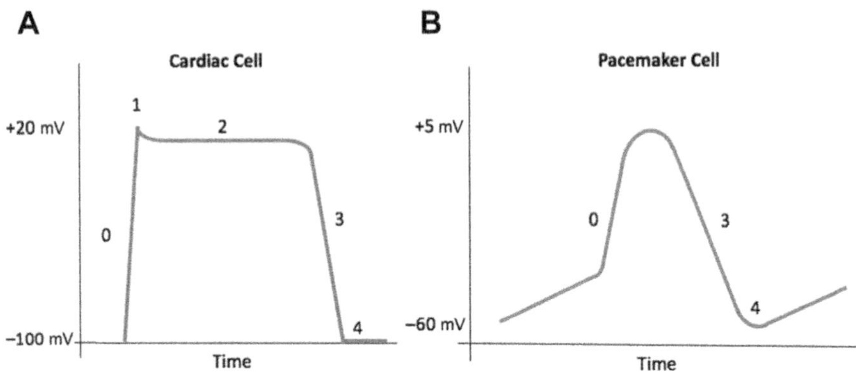

Fig. 2. (*A*) Normal cardiac cell action potential (*B*) pacemaker cell action potential. The action potential of pacemaker cells does not contain a plateau phase, allowing for a much more rapid contraction of the cell.

the cell cannot be stimulated again until it reaches its resting state. There are 2 stages to the refractory period: (1) the absolute refractory phase whereby no stimulation, no matter how great, will cause the cell to contract and (2) the relative refractory phase whereby a large enough electrical current will cause the cell to contract. These refractory phases prevent excessive, rapid contraction of a cardiac myocyte and results in stable and continuous propagation of the electrical current throughout the entire myocardium.

Action Potential of a Pacemaker Cell

Pacemaker cells, unlike standard cardiac myocytes, coordinate the rhythm and pace of the heartbeat and, therefore, have automaticity. All phases of depolarization and repolarization of a cardiac myocyte can be seen in **Fig. 2**B. Pacemaker cells are responsible for the generation of the cardiac impulse and, therefore, have a different action potential from that of standard, cardiac myocytes. Pacemaker cells do not actually contract and, therefore, have no plateau phase in their action potential.[7,10] The action potentials of pacemaker cells also differ from that of the normal, cardiac myocytes in that automatic cells have the ability to initiate an impulse or electrical current without any external stimulation.[11] In comparison, a normal cardiac myocyte can only contract when stimulated by an external impulse from an electrically coupled cell. The action potential of pacemaker cells is shown in comparison with the action potential of a normal cardiac cell in **Fig. 2**.

Ionic currents play a key role in the function of pacemaker cells. After repolarization, an outward current is created by potassium ions, which is, then, followed by an inward current of sodium ions. These sodium ions are activated after repolarization and are followed by a slow inward current of calcium ions, which are activated during depolarization of the cell membrane.[9,11]

Pacemaker cells are fundamental to the contraction of the heart and are found in 3 areas: the SA node, AV node, and bundle of His. Although the cells found in these areas are classified as automatic, the rate of depolarization does vary across all 3 types of automatic cells. The SA node has the shortest depolarization phase (phase 4) and, therefore, the quickest firing rate: approximately 60 to 100 times per minute. The AV junction has a lower firing rate of between 40 and 60 times per minutes; finally, the bundle branches and Purkinje fibers have a firing rate of less than 40 times per minute.[10]

THE CONDUCTION SYSTEM OF THE HEART

Possibly, the most important aspect of the contraction of the heart is the cardiac conduction system. The conduction system ensures that an electrical impulse generated by pacemaker cells in the SA node can effectively travel throughout the entire atrial and ventricular myocardium, creating a consistent and timely contraction of the heart muscle. The cardiac conduction system is composed of the SA node, the AV node, the bundle of His, bundle braches, and the Purkinje network. As mentioned previously, the heartbeat originates from the SA node in the upper right atrium and has the primary responsibility for the heart's electrical activity.

Atrial Activation

Atrial activation begins with the generation of a stimulating electrical impulse from the pacemaker cells of the SA node.[12] This pulse propagates freely throughout the atrial myocardium causing contraction of the right and left atria. Sir Thomas Lewis from the United Kingdom was the first to analyze contraction of the atria. He described it as follows:

> *...the excitation wave in the auricle may be likened to the spread of fluid poured upon a flat surface, it edges advancing as an ever widening circle, until the whole surface is covered; such variation as exists in the rate of travel along the varies lines in the auricle fully accounted for by the simple anatomical arrangement of the tissue.*
>
> *—Sir Thomas Lewis, 1908*[13]

The Sinoatrial Node

For years, many were baffled by how the heart beats until the electrical conduction system of the heart was fully accounted for by the discovery of the SA node by Keith and Flack in 1907.[12]

The SA node is a group of specialized myocardial cells located at the junction of the superior vena cava and the right atrium close to the crest of the atrial appendage. The node consists of 2 types of myocytes: (1) the central nodal cells, arranged in a complex interdigitating manner with connective tissue, and (2) the transitional myocytes that change gradually from the typical pacemaker cells to ordinary myocytes.[14]

The location of the SA node was first described by Lewis and colleagues[15] in 1910 and, later, confirmed on a canine model. In 1952, transmembrane potentials were first recorded from pacemaker cells of a frog heart.[14] This finding was closely followed by the mammalian heart in 1955.[16] These studies revealed that the most dominant feature of pacemaker cells is the spontaneous depolarization of the cell membrane. Further discoveries into the origin and function of pacemaker cells of the SA node occurred in 1963 when Trautwein and Uchizono[17] discovered dominant pacemaker cells in rabbits. They determined that the origin of the heartbeat occurred in a small area (approximately 0.3 mm^2), which contained about 5000 pacemaker cells that fire synchronously.[14]

Internodal Pathways

The impulse generated by pacemaker cells in the SA node is conducted through the atria via 4 main pathways in the atrium. Three of these pathways are found in the right atrium and one in the left atrium. These structures are known as internodal pathways as they carry the cardiac impulse from the SA node to the AV node. Internodal pathways consist of specialized myocytes, which run from the SA node to the AV node. Previously, internodal pathways were thought to consist of atrial myocytes alone; however, studies into the propagation speed of impulses from the SA node to the AV node found that the speed achieved was much greater than what is possible from normal atrial myocytes alone.[18] In fact, these internodal pathways have been shown to exhibit Purkinje fiberlike characteristics, meaning they have a much greater conduction velocity. However, much controversy still remains around this issue and the characteristics of the cells, which conduct the cardiac impulse from the SA node to the AV node have not been conclusively defined.[19] The conduction pathways for the cardiac impulse can be seen in **Fig. 3**.

VENTRICULAR ACTIVATION

The stimulus created by the SA node cannot be propagated throughout the ventricular myocardium because the atria and ventricles are separated by an electrically nonconductive cardiac skeleton. The AV node instead initiates contraction of the ventricular myocardium.

The Atrioventricular Node

The AV node coordinates the contraction of the heart by conducting the normal electrical impulse from the atria to the ventricles. The AV node delays the electrical impulse by approximately 0.12 s.[7] This delay is vital as it ensures the atria have filled with blood before the blood is ejected from the ventricles and pumped throughout the circulatory system. This delay ensures atrial-ventricular synchrony and allows for mechanical activity, which is far slower than electrical activity.

In the presence of atrial arrhythmias, such as atrial fibrillation (AF), the AV node is critically important because it actually blocks most of the many uncoordinated electrical impulses.[20] AV conduction during normal cardiac activation occurs via 2 different

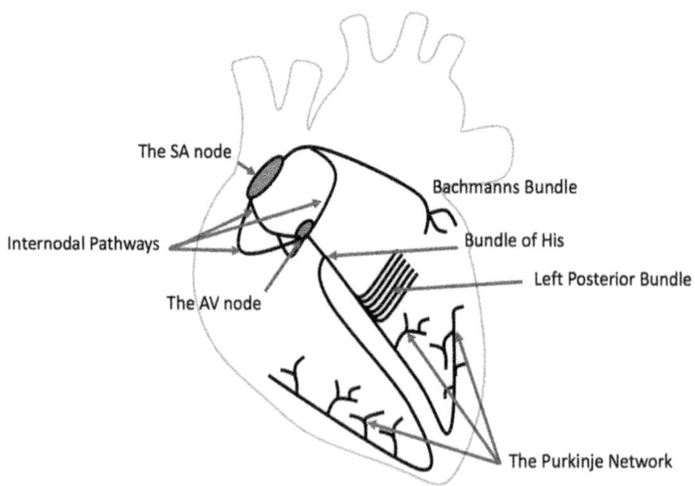

Fig. 3. The cardiac conduction system. Contraction of the heart begins at the SA node and is conducted to the AV node via intermodal pathways. From there the impulse is conducted through the ventricular myocardium via the Purkinje network.

pathways: (1) the first pathway has a slow conduction velocity but shorter refractory period and (2) the second pathway has a faster conduction velocity but longer refractory period.[14]

The Bundle of His, Bundle Branches, and the Purkinje Network

From the AV node the impulse is conducted to the bundle of His, which was discovered by Wilhelm His, a Swiss Cardiologist and Anatomist, in 1893.[10] The bundle of His is divided at the septum to provide the left and right bundle branches. These branches carry the cardiac impulse into both the left and right ventricles and end at a branching junction of the Purkinje system. The Purkinje system was discovered by the Czech physiologist Johannes Evangelist Purkinje in 1893. The primary function of the His-Purkinje system is to rapidly conduct the cardiac potential throughout the ventricles to ensure that the muscle contractions are in the correct order and blood is sufficiently ejected. The His-Purkinje system conducts action potentials much more rapidly than regular ventricular myocardium (2.3 m/s vs 0.75 m/s).[14]

FACTORS THAT INFLUENCE THE CARDIAC CONDUCTION SYSTEM

Autonomic Regulation

Because pacemaker cells within the cardiac conduction system have automaticity,[9] they do not require stimulation from the central nervous system. However, the heart is heavily influenced by the autonomic nervous system because sympathetic and parasympathetic nerve branches run from the brain to the heart.[21] These branches of nerves regulate heart rate, speed of conduction, and contractility, so that the heart can match cardiac output with the demands of the circulatory system during any given task. The sympathetic nerve supplies the SA node, AV node, atria, and ventricles and is responsible for the fight-or-flight complex.[7] Although not in detail here, but briefly put, the sympathetic nerve not only increases the heart rate but also alters the conduction and contractility of the heart. The sympathetic nerve has an increased activity during times of emotional excitement, exercise, and physiologic or psychological stress. For example, pharmaceuticals. such as beta-blockers, shield the heart from sympathetic nerve activity leading to a lower heart rate, blood pressure, and, as a result, a lower myocardial workload. The parasympathetic nerve supplies mainly the SA node and works in the opposite fashion as the sympathetic nervous system to slow down the heart. The more activity there is from the parasympathetic nerves, the slower the heart rate will become. Increased vagal tone is often associated with patients who suffer a myocardial infarction.

Abnormalities of the Conduction System

When there is damage to the normal conduction system of the heart, it can lead to severe clinical events. For example, patients suffering damage to the myocardium due to ischemic heart disease or bundle branch block can develop bradycardia[22] or defects, such as complete heart block. In addition, abnormal electrical conduction in the atrium, such as AF, is a leading cause of stroke events.[23,24] During AF the atria do not contract effectively, so blood begins to clot in the atria, particularly in the left atrial appendage.

Another example of abnormalities of the cardiac conduction stem is Wolff-Parkinson-White (WPW) syndrome. To maintain effective contraction of the myocardium, there must be a substantial delay between atrial and ventricular contraction (0.12 s). This delay allows the atria to complete its contraction and for the blood to effectively flow into and fill the ventricles. If this does not occur, which is the case in some patients with arrhythmias, such as WPW syndrome, there is a reduction in cardiac output.

THE CARDIAC CONDUCTION SYSTEM AND THE ELECTROCARDIOGRAM

The functioning of the cardiac conduction system can be recorded from the surface of the skin; this is known as the ECG. The ECG is a graphic representation of the electrical activity of the heart and is one of the most widely used diagnostic tools in medicine. As the ECG is a measurement of the electrical activity of the heart, it can be used to monitor and detect abnormalities in the normal cardiac conduction system. The ECG is recorded through conductive electrodes placed on the surface of the skin, which transduce the ionic current on the skin's surface to electrical current for analysis by electronic equipment.

In clinical practice, the most common device used to record the ECG is the 12-lead electrocardiograph,[25,26] which involves the placement of 10 electrodes on the body. Other ECG monitoring equipment, such as bedside monitors and telemetry systems, also record activity and supply data to analyze the ECG pattern. These methods of ECG monitoring are sometimes performed with a reduced number of electrodes, commonly 2 or 3. Analysis of the ECG is commonly performed via human

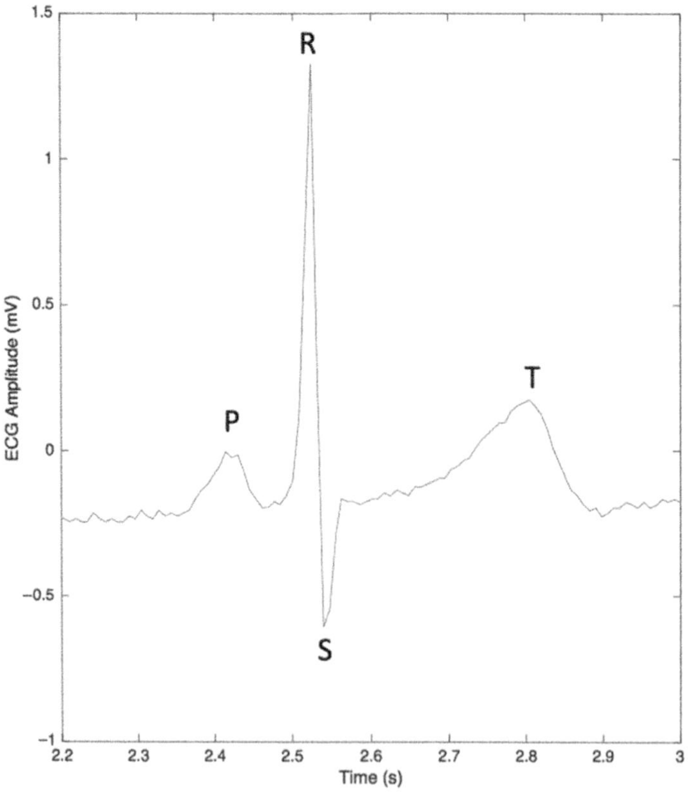

Fig. 4. A normal ECG waveform recorded from a healthy patient (16,272). This image outlines the key waveforms of a single-lead ECG recording from lead II. (*Adapted from* Goldberger AL, Amaral LA, Glass L, et al. PhysioBank, PhysioToolkit, and PhysioNet: components of a new research resource for complex physiologic signals. Circulation 2000;101:215–20.)

Table 1
Normal electrocardiogram wave and interval durations in relation to age

Parameter	Sex	Age (y) 16–19	20–29	30–39	40–49	50–59	60–69	70–79	80–89
Heart rate (beats per minute)	Male	73 (49; 107)	65 (45; 94)	65 (46; 95)	66 (47; 95)	67 (48; 94)	67 (48; 95)	67 (50; 99)	74 (40; 97)
	Female	72 (47; 105)	67 (48; 98)	66 (47; 95)	67 (47; 90)	69 (52; 94)	71 (53; 94)	72 (55; 98)	72 (50; 102)
P duration (ms)	Male	106 (90; 136)	110 (90; 128)	110 (90; 134)	110 (90; 134)	116 (94; 140)	120 (94; 146)	120 (94; 144)	121 (92; 152)
	Female	104 (89; 124)	104 (88; 122)	106 (89; 128)	108 (90; 128)	112 (92; 134)	114 (92; 138)	116 (90; 144)	118 (90; 146)
PQ duration (ms)	Male	148 (118; 200)	150 (118; 196)	152 (118; 198)	152 (115; 200)	160 (124; 206)	164 (126; 220)	164 (129; 228)	172 (122; 290)
	Female	144 (112; 190)	144 (110; 190)	146 (114; 196)	148 (112; 200)	156 (120; 206)	158 (120; 206)	162 (121; 210)	170 (125; 235)
QRS duration (ms)	Male	100 (82; 126)	100 (80; 126)	100 (78; 124)	100 (78; 122)	100 (80; 124)	100 (80; 124)	101 (80; 131)	98 (70; 136)
	Female	92 (74; 112)	90 (76; 110)	92 (74; 114)	90 (76; 114)	92 (76; 114)	92 (76; 115)	92 (74; 114)	92 (72; 118)
QT interval (ms)	Male	378 (332; 452)	394 (342; 454)	396 (344; 454)	394 (342; 458)	396 (342; 458)	398 (346; 454)	398 (336; 458)	395 (334; 476)
	Female	390 (337; 455)	394 (340; 456)	400 (346; 460)	396 (350; 458)	398 (349; 458)	396 (351; 454)	394 (342; 454)	394 (332; 461)

Values represent median (2nd percentile; 98th percentile).

Data from Rijnbeek PR, van Herpen G, Bots ML, et al. Normal values of the electrocardiogram for ages 16-90 years. J Electrocardiol 2014;47(6):914–21.

interpretation[27]; however; some ECG monitoring systems provide automated arrhythmia analysis.

The ECG consists of 5 main wave characteristics known as the PQRST complex, as shown in **Fig. 4**. The P wave reflects atrial depolarization (contraction). The P-Q interval is referred to as the period of atrial systole, which corresponds to the time it takes for the impulse to travel from the SA node to the AV node via the internodal pathways. The QRS complex refers to the conduction of the cardiac impulse through the AV node, the bundle of His, the bundle branches, and the Purkinje network and, therefore, represents depolarization of the ventricular myocardium. The T wave represents repolarization of the ventricular myocardium whereby all cardiac cells return to their resting potential and the completion the heartbeat is achieved.

Table 1 shows normal values for heartbeat and waveform intervals for both males and females across different age groups; interestingly, all intervals remain consistent across age groups except for the PQ interval, which increased in duration with age.

SUMMARY

The normal conduction system of the heart is a complex structure composed of specialized cells, which allow for spontaneous initiation and conduction of an electrical impulse. These impulses are responsible for the contraction of the myocardium in a synchronized fashion and the maintenance of an adequate heart rate. However, if abnormalities are found in any of the components of the cardiac conduction system, this can lead to dangerous heart rates and rhythms.

A fundamental principle of contraction of the heart is the spontaneous generation of an electrical impulse, which occurs because of rapid changes in the permeability of the pacemaker cells. This electrical impulse is generated from pacemaker's cells, found in the SA node that is responsible for atrial activation. The impulse is then conducted to the AV node through internodal pathways. The impulse then enters the bundle of His where it is conducted to the Purkinje network, and the complete contraction of the heart muscle is achieved.

The key components of the cardiac conduction system and how these components function together to allow for normal and sustained beating of the heart have been described. Some abnormalities that can be found in the cardiac conduction system due to cardiovascular disease have also been briefly outlined. Understanding the key principles discussed and knowing how they relate to the origin and maintenance of the heartbeat should allow for a better understanding of the underlying physiology of the heart, leading to a better grasp of more complex pathologies.

REFERENCES

1. Mahmood SS, Levy D, Vasan RS, et al. The Framingham Heart Study and the epidemiology of cardiovascular disease: a historical perspective. Lancet 2014; 383(9921):999–1008.
2. Allender S, Scarborough P, Peto V, et al. European cardiovascular disease statistics. 3rd edition. Brussels (Belgium): A Eur Hear NetworkEuropean Hear Netw; 2008. p. 1773.
3. Park DS, Fishman GI. The cardiac conduction system. Circulation 2011;123(8): 904–15.
4. Dhein S. Cardiac gap junctions. Physiol Regul Pathophysiol Pharmacol 1998.
5. Tortora GJ, Nielsen MT. Principles of human anatomy. 13th edition. Hoboken (NJ): Wiley; 2014.

6. Alberts B, Bray D, Hopkin K, et al. Essential cell biology. New York: Garland Science; 2013.
7. Sampson M, McGrath A. Understanding the ECG. Part 1: anatomy and physiology. Br J Card Nurs 2015;10(11):548–54.
8. Roden DM, Balser JR, George AL Jr, et al. Cardiac ion channels. Annu Rev Physiol 2002;64(1):431–75.
9. Grant AO. Cardiac ion channels. Circ Arrhythm Electrophysiol 2009;2(2):185–94.
10. Jevon P. ECGs for nurses, vol. 14. New Jersey: John Wiley & Sons; 2009.
11. DiFrancesco D. Pacemaker mechanisms in cardiac tissue. Annu Rev Physiol 1993;55(1):455–72.
12. Silverman ME, Hollman A. Discovery of the sinus node by Keith and Flack: on the centennial of their 1907 publication. Heart 2007;93(10):1184–7.
13. Lewis T. Lectures on the heart. PB Hoeber; 1915.
14. Macfarlane PW, van Oosterom A, Pahlm O, et al, editors. Comprehensive electrocardiology. 2nd edition. Vol. 1. Springer; 2011. p. 391–3.
15. Lewis T, Oppenheimer BS, Oppenheimer A. The site of origin of the mammalian heartbeat: the pacemaker in the dog. Heart 1910;2(147):1910–1.
16. WEST TC. Ultramicroelectrode recording from the cardiac pacemaker. J Pharmacol Exp Ther 1955;115(3):283–90.
17. Trautwein W, Uchizono K. Electron microscopic and electrophysiologic study of the pacemaker in the sino-atrial node of the rabbit heart. Z Zellforsch Mikrosk Anat 1963;61(1):96–109.
18. Anderson RH, Ho SY, Smith A, et al. The internodal atrial myocardium. Anat Rec 1981;201(1):75–82.
19. Kafer CJ. Internodal pathways in the human atria: a model study. Comput Biomed Res 1991;24(6):549–63.
20. Mainardi L, Sornmo L, Cerutti S. Understanding atrial fibrillation: the signal processing contribution. California: Morgan & Claypool Publishers; 2008.
21. Ekman P, Levenson RW, Friesen WV. Autonomic nervous system activity distinguishes among emotions. Science 1983;221(4616):1208–10.
22. Grauer LE, Gershen BJ, Orlando MM, et al. Bradycardia and its complications in the prehospital phase of acute myocardial infarction. Am J Cardiol 1973;32(5):607–11.
23. Gladstone DJ, Spring M, Dorian P, et al. Atrial fibrillation in patients with cryptogenic stroke. N Engl J Med 2014;370(26):2467–77.
24. Gladstone DJ, Bui E, Fang J, et al. Potentially preventable strokes in high-risk patients with atrial fibrillation who are not adequately anticoagulated. Stroke 2009;40(1):235–40.
25. Kennedy A, Finlay DD, Guldenring D, et al. Improved recording of atrial activity by modified bipolar leads derived from the 12-lead electrocardiogram. J Electrocardiol 2015;48(6):1017–21.
26. Finlay DD, Nugent CD, Kellett JG, et al. Synthesising the 12-lead electrocardiogram: trends and challenges. Eur J Intern Med 2007;18(8):566–70.
27. Bond RR, Finlay DD, Breen C, et al. Eye tracking in the assessment of electrocardiogram interpretation techniques. Comput Cardiol 2012;39:581–4. Available at: http://www.scopus.com/inward/record.url?eid=2-s2.0-84875666610&partnerID=tZOtx3y1.

The Normal Electrocardiogram

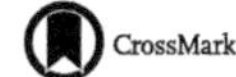

Resting 12-Lead and Electrocardiogram Monitoring in the Hospital

Patricia R.E. Harris, PhD, RN, CNS

KEYWORDS

• Cardiac rhythm • Electrocardiography • Electrocardiogram • 12-lead ECG
• Cardiac monitoring

KEY POINTS

- Cardiac rhythm assessment is a diagnostic tool providing health care clinicians with vital information about their patients' physiologic conditions.
- Mastery of electrocardiographic monitoring and competent interpretation of patients' cardiovascular responses are essential components of the critical care nurse's clinical knowledge repertoire.
- In intensive care, goals of electrocardiographic monitoring include detection of:
  - Cardiac ischemia.
  - Arrhythmias.
  - QT interval changes.
- Future directions for electrocardiographic monitoring may include more accurate beat detection and improved predictive models.

INTRODUCTION OF THE ELECTROCARDIOGRAPH

Electrocardiography has been described as one of the greatest developments in cardiovascular science of the twentieth century,[1] and electrocardiographic monitoring is a standard of practice in critical care units throughout the United States.[2] Knowledge of electrocardiography and accurate interpretation of cardiac rhythm provides vital information about patients' dynamic physiologic conditions.[3] Over the last 50 years, a thorough education and a detailed knowledge of electrocardiographic features, along with patients' cardiovascular responses, have become essential tools of critical care nurses.[4–6]

Disclosure: The author has nothing to disclose.
Department of Nursing, School of Health and Natural Sciences, Dominican University of California, 50 Acacia Avenue, San Rafael, CA 94901, USA
E-mail address: patricia.harris@dominican.edu

Crit Care Nurs Clin N Am 28 (2016) 281–296
http://dx.doi.org/10.1016/j.cnc.2016.04.002 ccnursing.theclinics.com
0899-5885/16/$ – see front matter © 2016 Elsevier Inc. All rights reserved.

Historical Highlights

In 1786, Italian scientist Luigi Galvani studied the effect of electricity on animal muscle. He found that direct contact with an electrical generator led to muscular contraction, and he explained his findings in terms of "animal electricity." His experimentation in this field led him to discover that electrical stimulation of a frog's heart is associated with cardiac muscular contraction.[7]

In 1856, 2 physiologists, Albert Kölliker from Switzerland and Heinrich Müller from Germany, using a galvanometer devised to measure a small amount of electrical current and named for Galvani, showed that the heart produced electrical activity, corresponding with each contraction of the heart.[8,9]

The French-born and Scottish-trained physician Augustus Waller[11] first correlated electrocardiographic signals with the human heartbeat in 1887.[10] During his appointment as professor of physiology at St Mary's Hospital in the United Kingdom, he conceptualized an experiment to record the electrical activity of the human heart. Using zinc electrodes and a device called a capillary electrometer, he was able to record the world's first human electrocardiogram (ECG), which he subsequently published. In his publication, Waller[11] also described the variations in the electrical signal recording that arose from changes in electrode placement,[10,11] a phenomenon with which present day intensive care nurses are familiar.[12,13]

Dutch physiologist Willem Einthoven witnessed a demonstration of the electrometer by Waller, recording the heart's electrical activity, and was inspired. Dr Einthoven's groundbreaking work, using the string galvanometer, a refined version of the earlier galvanometer, to measure the electrical activity of the heart, advanced the science of cardiology. He was the first to call the recording device an electrocardiograph and the resulting recording an ECG (also abbreviated EKG for the German spelling of elektrokardiografi). He was awarded the Nobel Prize for his contribution to cardiovascular physiology in 1924.[6,14,15]

Ubiquitous Use in Modern Intensive Care

Introduced in coronary care units during the 1960s, electrocardiography has become crucial for early recognition of changes in patients' complex conditions.[4,5,16] The ECG is now among the most commonly conducted diagnostic tool, and it remains a fundamental tool of clinical practice for assessment of cardiovascular health.[17] ECG technology continues to evolve, so competent interpretation of the electrocardiographic waveforms is an essential skill for critical care nurses and other clinicians.[2,3,18]

THE NORMAL RESTING 12-LEAD ELECTROCARDIOGRAM

The standard 12-lead ECG provides a graphic representation of the myocardium's electrical activity, recorded from 12 different views with 10 surface electrodes.[2,17] The electrodes detect variations in electrical potential caused by the excitation of the myocardium so that measurement of the amplitude and duration of the waveforms can be calculated.[19,20]

Orientation to the Resting 12-lead Electrocardiogram

Typically, the 12-lead ECG printout contains the patient's identifying information, such as name, medical record number, gender, age, and/or birth date. Measurements, computed by the software algorithm, typically include heart rate and waveform intervals: PR interval, QRS complex, QT/corrected QT (QTc) interval, QRS axis, and interpretation of the cardiac rhythm. Other information at the bottom of the 12-lead ECG includes calibrations, the paper speed of 25 mm/s on the horizontal axis; the sensitivity setting of 10 mm/mV, and the filter's frequency setting to reduce artifact (150 Hz) (**Fig. 1**).

The vertical block at the beginning of each row shows the calibration mark, which is an amplitude of 1 mV signal. The height of these signals are measurements of voltage, and the standard setting is 10 mm per 1 mV.[19] The main body of the record depicts the electrocardiographic waveforms. The ECG graph paper produces a record of time on the horizontal axis, measured in seconds or milliseconds. The graph is divided into boxes with each large box containing 25 smaller boxes: 5 on the horizontal axis and 5 on the vertical axis. On the horizontal axis, each small horizontal box is 0.04 seconds and each large box is 0.20 seconds in duration. Consequently, 5 large boxes equal 1 second, 15 large boxes are equal to 3 seconds, and 30 large boxes equal 6 seconds. The vertical axis depicts amplitude in millimeters or voltage in millivolts.[18,19]

Three major properties of cardiac muscle can be evaluated with the ECG: automaticity, conductivity, and excitability or irritability.[20]

- Automaticity refers to the ability of the pacemaker to initiate an electrical impulse, an effect of chronotropy. The impact of changes in heart rate, the chronotropic response, has important implications for cardiac function and for patients' quality of life.[21]
- Conductivity refers to the ability of the cardiac myocytes to conduct an electrical impulse, an effect of dromotropy. The cardiac electrical conduction system refers to a group of specialized cardiac myocytes that signal the myocardium to contract. The normal activation sequence of the cardiac conduction system starts with an impulse in the sinoatrial node, initiating a wave of depolarization through the atrial myocardium to the atrioventricular node. The wave of depolarization moves through the ventricles via the bundle of His, right and left bundle branches, and Purkinje fibers.[21,22]
- Irritability or excitability refers to the ability of the myocyte to respond to a stimulus. The effect of this stimulation is called bathmotropy. The electrical stimulus required to consistently elicit a cardiac depolarization is expressed in terms of amplitude (volts or milliamps), pulse width (milliseconds), and energy (microjoules).[21]

As Kölliker and Müller showed, with each heartbeat, an electrical impulse travels through the heart, generating a wave.[9] In normal cardiac physiology, 1 heartbeat corresponds with the timing of the electrical activity that travels through the atrium and ventricles. The wave therefore corresponds with the mechanical cardiac muscular contraction and propulsion of blood from the heart.[22]

ELECTRODES AND LEADS

In ECG terminology, the word lead can refer to the wires that connect to the electrode or to a graphic representation of the electrical activity of the heart at the heart's surface.[22]

Standard Electrode Placement

Ten electrodes are placed on the body surface to generate 12 different views of the heart's electrical activity.[2,17] Placement of electrodes is shown in **Box 1**.

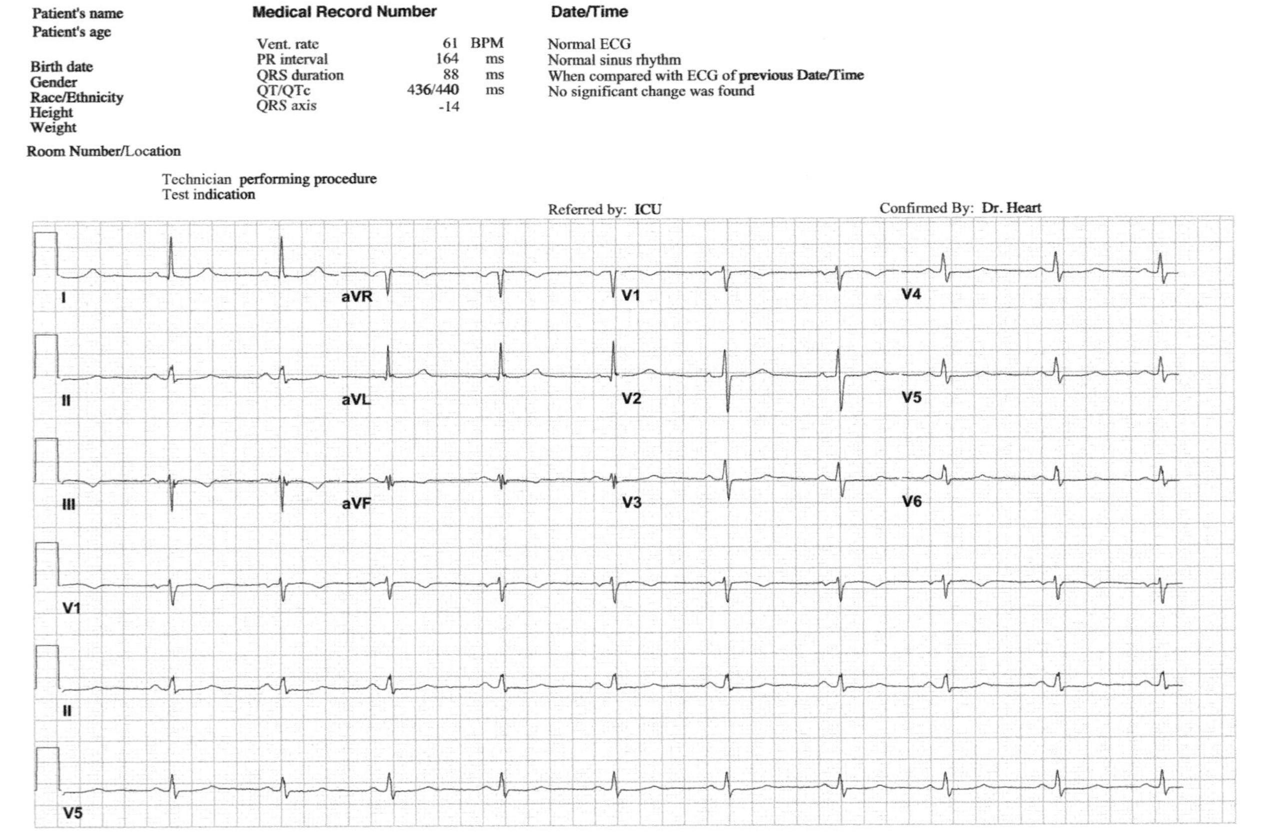

Fig. 1. Normal resting electrocardiogram. aVF, augmented vector foot; aVL, augmented vector left; aVR, augmented vector right.

Box 1
Placement of limb and chest lead

Four limb electrodes

- Left arm (LA): distal left arm
- Right arm (RA): distal right arm
- Right leg (RL): reference or ground lead, usually placed on distal right leg
- Left leg (LL): distal left leg

Six chest electrodes

- V1: placed in the fourth intercostal space, right of the sternum
- V2: placed in the fourth intercostal space, left of the sternum
- V3: placed between V2 and V4
- V4: placed at the fifth intercostal space in the nipple line; under the breast in women
- V5: placed between V4 and V6
- V6: placed in the midaxillary line on the same height as V4 (horizontal line from V4)

Data from Refs.[17–19]

Patient and Skin Preparation

Proper electrode placement requires preparation of the skin to help reduce signal noise and potential artifact. Recommendations include cleansing the skin with mild soap and water or alcohol to remove skin oils and debris before electrode placement. Wiping the area with a rough washcloth, gauze, or a light sandpaper to roughen the skin may help reduce skin impedance. Clipping excess hair at the electrode site is also recommended.[23]

Spatial Orientation

Each of the 12 leads represents a particular orientation in space.[18,19] The 12-lead ECG provides spatial information about cardiac electrical activity in 3 intersecting directions. These are:

- Anterior ↔ posterior, crossing the frontal (or coronal) plane
- Superior ↔ inferior, crossing the horizontal (or transverse) plane
- Right ↔ left, crossing the sagittal plane

Polarity

The conventional standard ECG lead system changes polarity according to the internal programming of the electrocardiograph. This change in polarity affects the electrodes that are placed in the positions of right arm, left arm, and left leg. The right leg serves as a reference lead, and is used as a neutral or zero point, from which electrical current is measured.[22]

Standard Leads

Besides introducing the world to the ECG, Einthoven established the foundation of ECG analysis with the presentation of the Einthoven triangle.

Standard limb leads include leads I, II, and III, and record electrical activity over the frontal plane of the thorax, and are place approximately equidistant from the center of the heart's electrical activity. Leads I, II, and III record the electrical potential between 2 electrodes also known as bipolar leads.[19]

In the configuration for lead I, the positive electrode is on the left arm, and the negative electrode on the right arm, measuring the difference in electrical potential between the two arms. In the lead II configuration, the positive electrode is on the left leg and the negative electrode is on the right arm. Lead III has the positive electrode on the left leg and the negative electrode on the left arm.[18,19]

These 3 bipolar limb leads roughly form an equilateral triangle with the heart at the center; hence, Einthoven triangle.[24] Bipolar refers to 1 electrode being defined as the positive pole, whereas the second electrode provides the negative pole. Limb leads can be attached to the distal end of a limb (ankles and wrists) or near the proximal end of a limb (hips or upper thighs and shoulders). When placing limb electrodes, uniformity is important. For example, 2 electrodes belong on the shoulders or 2 on the wrists, not 1 electrode on a wrist and the other on a shoulder. In addition, the electrodes must be consistently placed in the same location for sequential ECGs.[2,17,22]

Augmented Leads

The augmented leads, augmented vector right (aVR), augmented vector left (aVL), and augmented vector foot (aVF), are computer derived to provide clinicians with additional information. The augmented leads use the same electrodes as the standard limb leads, but the leads are unipolar and view the heart from different aspects across the frontal plane. In unipolar leads, electrical current that flows toward an electrode produces a positive deflection (upward), whereas current receding from the electrode produces a negative deflection (downward). The term augmented refers to the amplitude of the signal in these leads, which is increased by 50%. Lead aVR provides visualization of the heart from the viewpoint of the right shoulder, lead aVL provides visualization of the heart from the left shoulder or primarily a view of the left ventricle wall, and lead aVF provides visualization of the heart from the viewpoint of the lower limb or foot to view the heart's inferior surface (**Fig. 2**).[17,19]

Chest Leads

Leads V_1 to V_6 are the chest leads and view from the transverse or horizontal plane of the heart. Like the augmented leads, these are unipolar leads. Along with inferior and superior views of the heart, the 6 chest leads allow visualization of the anterior and posterior surfaces of the heart.[17,19]

Mason-Likar Lead Placement

From 1964 to 1966, cardiologists and medical researchers Robert E. Mason and Ivan Likar experimented with electrode placement and introduced the modified 12-lead ECG, now called the Mason-Likar system.[25,26] The Mason-Likar system was designed to reduce muscle artifact from limb movement during exercise stress testing. Changing the placement of the right arm (RA) and left arm (LA) electrodes to the infraclavicular fossa medial to the border of the deltoid muscle and 2 cm below the lower border of the clavicle provided recordings with less noise while maintaining waveform morphology similar to the presentation of waveforms recorded with electrodes placed on the extremities; the left leg (LL) electrode was moved to "the anterior axillary line, halfway between the costal margin and the crest of the ilium".[26(p198)] The researchers noted that the precise position of LL was less crucial than RA or LA in maintaining adequate noise reduction along with waveforms similar to those produced by electrodes placed on the extremity and could be varied by a few centimeters. The right

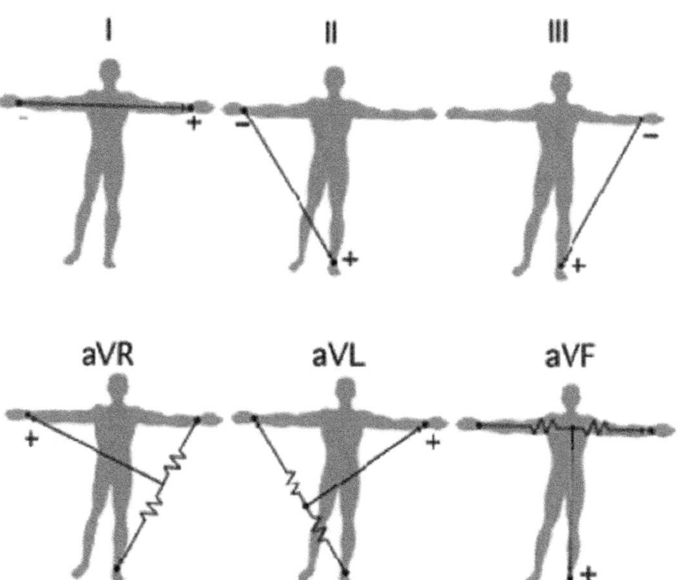

Fig. 2. The Einthoven triangle with standard and augmented ECG leads. The standard leads are placed on the right arm, left arm, and left leg and record the heart's electrical activity in the frontal plane. The same electrodes that record electrical activity for the limb leads are used for the unipolar augmented leads. The augmented leads measure the electrical potential at 1 point with respect to a null point that does not register electrical potential and is determined for each lead by adding the potential from the other 2 leads. (*From* Nobelprize.org. The electrocardiogram, ECG. 2014. Available at: http://www.nobelprize.org/educational/medicine/ecg/ecg-readmore.htm. Accessed December 9, 2015; with permission.)

leg (RL) or reference electrode, usually is situated opposite the LL electrode, on the right iliac fossa (**Fig. 3**).[2]

Electrocardiogram Waves and Time Intervals

The normal ECG is composed of the P wave, QRS complex, T wave, and, possibly, a U wave (**Fig. 4**).[17,19,27]

The contraction of the right and left atria corresponds with the first wave, called the P wave, followed by an isoelectric line, as the electrical impulse travels to the ventricles. The contraction of the right and left ventricles corresponds with the QRS complex, followed by the T wave representing electrical recovery; that is, ventricular repolarization, or return to a resting state of the ventricles. If present, the U wave, a normal variant that follows the T wave, is associated with slow heart rates (<65 beats per minute), and may represent an after-repolarization phenomenon at the beginning of diastole.[19,27]

Sinus Rhythm

In healthy individuals, sinus rhythm should be the dominant cardiac rhythm, and has several key ECG features (**Box 2**).

There can be a wide range of normal in the ECG with regard to ECG features, and **Table 1** provides a framework, but there may be normal variations that diverge from these reference values. In particular, values can change according to age and sex.[27]

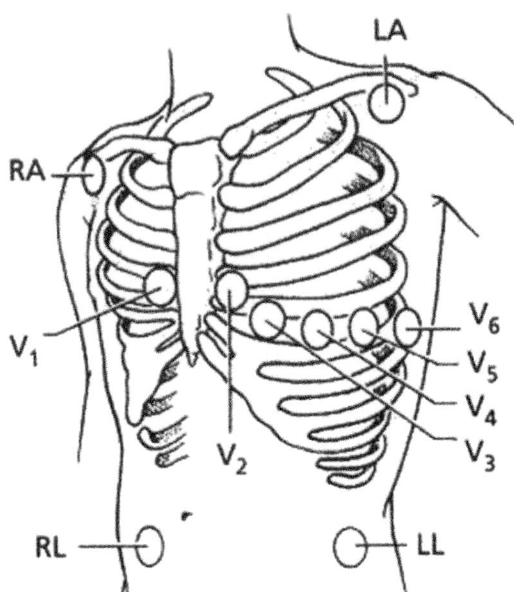

Fig. 3. The Mason-Likar electrode placement for continuous 12-lead monitoring. (*From* Drew BJ, Califf RM, Funk M, et al. Practice standards for electrocardiographic monitoring in hospital settings: an American Heart Association scientific statement from the Councils on Cardiovascular Nursing, Clinical Cardiology, and Cardiovascular Disease in the Young: endorsed by the International Society of Computerized Electrocardiology and the American Association of Critical-Care Nurses. Circulation 2004;110(17):2721–46; with permission.)

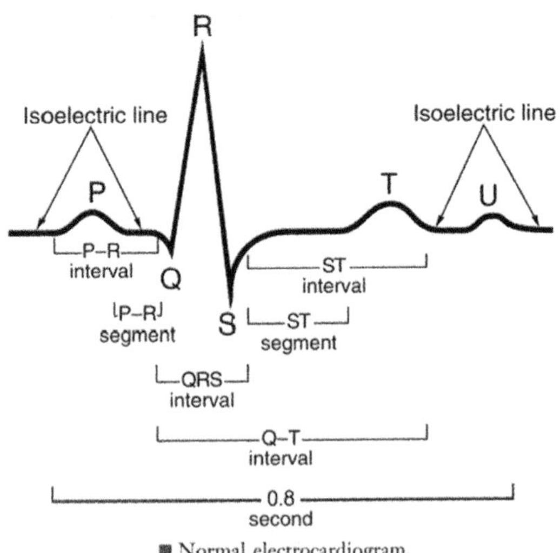

Fig. 4. Normal ECG cycle in lead I. (*From* Yanowitz F. Introduction to ECG interpretation: the standard 12-lead ECG 2012; ECG Learning Center dedicated to Alan E. Lindsay. Available at: http://ecg.utah.edu/. Accessed May 11, 2016.)

Box 2
Identification of sinus rhythm

- There is a P wave before each QRS complex
- P waves in leads I and II are upright (positive)
- P waves are rounded and uniform in shape
- The PR interval is fixed and within the normal duration range
- Rhythm needs to be regular[19,22]

Data from Yanowitz F. Introduction to ECG interpretation: The standard 12-lead ECG 2012; ECG Learning Center dedicated to Alan E. Lindsay. Available at: http://ecg.utah.edu/. Accessed May 11, 2016; and Goldberger AL. Introductory principles clinical electrocardiography: a simplified approach. 7th edition. Philadelphia: Mosby; 2006. p. 3–6.

Table 1
Normal ECG features, action, and reference duration in adults

ECG Feature	Action	Normal Duration
P wave	Depolarization of the right and left atria	0.08–0.11 s[29]
PR interval	Onset of atrial depolarization (P wave) to onset of ventricular depolarization (start of QRS complex)	0.12–0.20 s[29]
Q wave	First negative deflection after the P wave, if present	<0.04 s with depth of less than one-quarter of R wave amplitude[29]
QRS complex	Right and left ventricular depolarization	0.07–0.10 s[29]
J point	Junction between the end of the T wave and the beginning of the ST segment	Not applicable
U wave	Low-frequency deflection that occurs after the T wave. May represent an after-repolarization phase of ventricles	Bradycardia may enhance the U-wave amplitude; rarely present at rates >95 beats per minute[29]
QT interval	Duration of ventricular depolarization and repolarization; measured from the beginning of the QRS complex to end of T wave	Heart rate dependent; decreases with increasing heart rate[30]
QTc	Rate-corrected QT interval. Two frequently used nonlinear formulas computed with RR interval in seconds • Bazett: QTc = QT/√RR[31] • Fridericia: QTc = QT/3√RR[31] One linear formula with RR interval is in milliseconds. • Framingham: QTc = QT + 0.154 (1-RR)[30]	Typical normal values: <0.46 in men[29] <0.47 in women[29] QTc >500 ms is associated with an increased risk of torsades de pointes

Data from Refs.[19,28–31]

Waveform Deflection

The ECG tracing consists of numerous waveforms and intervals all carefully labeled to provide ECG nomenclature so that clinicians are able to communicate about the waveform to other clinicians. For example, a clinician may ask, "Do you see the development of new Q waves?" Thus, for the QRS complex, Q and S waves are always negative and the R wave is always positive.[18]

In the frontal plane view, the normal QRS complex appears upright and positive in leads I, II, III, aVL, and aVF. The only limb lead with an electrode on the right side of the body is aVR. The positive electrode is located on the right arm and visualizes the area to the left and downward. This direction is the same as that in which the electrical current flows, away from the positive electrode for lead aVR, thus generating a negative deflection.[19]

In the horizontal plane, the R-wave deflections in the V leads move progressively from being very short in V_1 to very tall in V_5. The R wave in V_6 remains tall. This phenomenon of R-wave progression occurs because the electrical current flows toward the positive electrode of V_4.[18,19] In the horizontal plane view, the normal QRS complex deflects downward in lead V_1 and V_2.[18]

Both limb and precordial lead waveforms cross the sagittal plane (plane spanning right to left or vice versa).

QRS Axis

The QRS axis refers to the direction in which the mean QRS vector current flows in the frontal plane. The normal axis points mostly downward and to the left because the more muscular left ventricle generates a stronger depolarizing current, which overwhelms that generated by the less bulky right.[17,19]

The normal QRS axis is between −30° and +90°. One simple way to estimate the ECG axis is to check the deflection of the QRS complex in leads I and aVF. The normal QRS complex is positive in both lead I and lead aVF; thus, if these leads are positive, this indicates that the axis is within the normal range.[19,20]

Electrocardiogram Case Study

Mr J is a 50-year-old man who was playing softball when he slid into second base and severely twisted his ankle. In the emergency department, a radiological study revealed that he had sustained a fractured fibula and would require a surgical repair with open reduction internal fixation. As a precaution before the surgical procedure, a resting 12-lead ECG was obtained (**Fig. 5**). The ECG showed normal sinus rhythm at 63 beats per minute; leads I and aVF deflecting upward, indicating that the QRS axis was within the normal range; and all of the interval measures were within normal ranges; thus he was cleared for surgery.

CONTINUOUS ELECTROCARDIOGRAM MONITORING IN THE HOSPITAL

Overview of Electrocardiogram Monitoring in Intensive Care

Specialized coronary care units were first introduced to advance the care of patients with myocardial infarction during the early 1960s.[5,6,16] The need for continuous electrocardiographic monitoring expanded as lifesaving treatments, such as the ability to safely defibrillate patients with lethal arrhythmias, became the standard of care.[31] Well-trained clinicians who are able to recognize subtle changes in cardiac rhythm along with the associated physiological changes, are essential for the provision of high quality coronary care.[32]

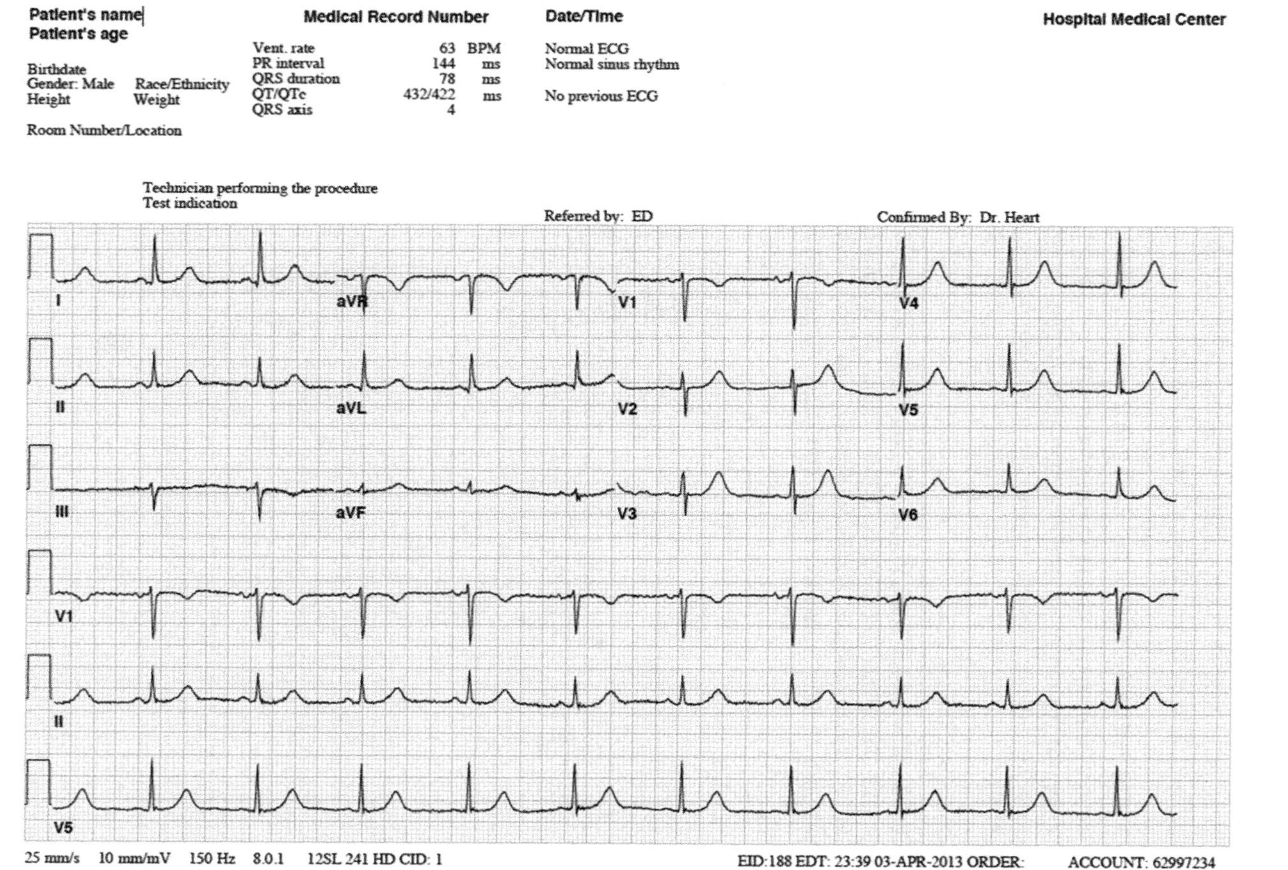

Fig. 5. Case study: Mr J's 12-lead ECG.

ECG monitoring is recommended for a wide range of patient conditions.[2,16] In addition to patients with known cardiac risk factors, such as having a diagnosis of diabetes,[33] monitoring may be needed for those patients admitted to intensive care with sepsis and shock,[34] respiratory dysfunction,[35] trauma,[36] acute renal failure,[37] cerebrovascular disorders such as stroke,[2] drug overdose (especially from known arrhythmogenic drugs),[2,38] and major noncardiac surgery (especially in older adult patients with coronary artery disease risk factors).[2]

Lead Configuration for Continuous Monitoring

The Mason-Likar electrode configuration is widely used in intensive care settings, and serves to reduce noise during continuous cardiac monitoring. A 5-electrode system is commonly used to record the limb leads and 1 precordial or V lead (**Fig. 6**).[2]

Indications for Monitoring

The American Heart Association, Councils on Cardiovascular Nursing, Clinical Cardiology, and Cardiovascular Disease in the Young, all endorsed by the International Society of Computerized Electrocardiology and the American Association of Critical-Care Nurses, published a position paper to provide recommendations for

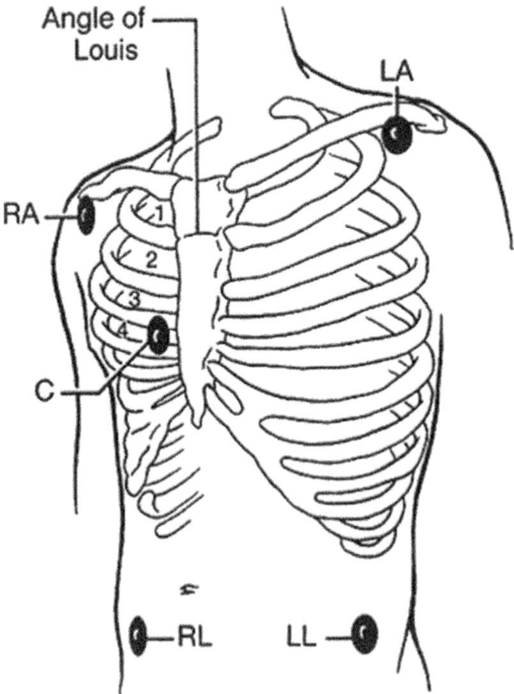

Fig. 6. The Mason-Likar electrode placement for continuous bedside monitoring. (*From* Drew BJ, Califf RM, Funk M, et al. Practice standards for electrocardiographic monitoring in hospital settings: an American Heart Association scientific statement from the Councils on Cardiovascular Nursing, Clinical Cardiology, and Cardiovascular Disease in the Young: endorsed by the International Society of Computerized Electrocardiology and the American Association of Critical-Care Nurses. Circulation 2004;110(17):2721–46; with permission.)

best practices in hospital ECG monitoring for adults and children, including ST segment and ischemia, arrhythmia, and QT interval monitoring for children and adults. Three important goals of cardiac monitoring are detection of ischemia, detection of arrhythmias, and prolongation of the QT interval[2] (**Box 3**).

Skills and Responsibilities for Monitoring

Knowledge of the indications and goals for continuous monitoring, of procedures for skin preparation, and of correct electrode placement, and knowledge of interpretation of normal ECG findings is essential for intensive care nurses.[39] Nurses are responsible for vigilantly monitoring changes in ECG waveforms, maintaining awareness of patients' physiologic responses to these changes, and intervening when necessary.[3,31,32]

The physiologic monitor's computer algorithms have been designed to be very sensitive, providing precise information about changes in the heart's electrical activity. Detection of any deviation from the patient's electrocardiographic baseline is paramount. However, sensitivity has been emphasized more than specificity, resulting in frequent detection of conditions that are not abnormal, and thus are not actionable.[39] Intensive care nurses must be ready to evaluate their patients, to identify true abnormalities, and be ready to respond to true cardiac events in good nursing. Recognition of what constitutes normal is the first step.

Box 3
Goals of continuous cardiac monitoring in critical care

Ischemia ST segment monitoring

- Monitoring for ST segment elevation or depression is indicated for patients who are admitted with acute coronary syndrome, and patients recovering from cardiopulmonary resuscitation or cardiac surgery. In addition, patients diagnosed with sepsis, shock, respiratory failure, and acute kidney injury are at high risk for ischemic episodes.[2]

Arrhythmia monitoring

- Arrhythmia monitoring is indicated for all patients entering the critical care unit. Among those with indications for continuous monitoring are patients who may not necessarily be diagnosed with preexisting cardiovascular conditions.[24] Patients at risk for experiencing arrhythmic events may be similar to those for ischemia.[2]

QT interval monitoring

- The QT interval is considered to be a surrogate measure of ventricular repolarization. The QT interval measurement needs to be corrected for heart rate, using one of the common formulas, to be considered accurate. QT prolongation has been associated with increased incidences of the polymorphic dysrhythmia torsades de pointes. Therefore, QT monitoring is indicated for any patient with increased risk for long QT, including patients with administered proarrhythmic medications known to increase the risk for torsades de pointes.

Data from Drew BJ, Califf RM, Funk M, et al. Practice standards for electrocardiographic monitoring in hospital settings: an American Heart Association scientific statement from the Councils on Cardiovascular Nursing, Clinical Cardiology, and Cardiovascular Disease in the Young: endorsed by the International Society of Computerized Electrocardiology and the American Association of Critical-Care Nurses. Circulation 2004;110(17):2721–46; and Moss AJ, Wojciech Zareba C, Benhorin J, et al. ISHNE guidelines for electrocardiographic evaluation of drug-related QT prolongation and other alterations in ventricular repolarization: task force summary. A report of the Task Force of the International Society for Holter and Noninvasive Electrocardiology (ISHNE), Committee on Ventricular Repolarization. Ann Noninvasive Electrocardiol 2001;6(4):333–41.

FUTURE DIRECTIONS

Advances in computerized electrocardiography include development of accurate algorithms,[40] potentially increasing specificity; for example, the recognition of events that are not true, while maintaining high sensitivity to the recognition of events that are true.[41]

Future directions for electrocardiography include automated detection of misplaced electrodes[42]; improved predictive models for acute cardiac events[43,44]; refinement of distinctions for age, gender, race,[45] and genetics[46]; development of accurate surrogate measures for cardiac autonomic function[47] and respiratory activity[48]; and increased security as ECG data move to cloud computing.[49] The need for critical care nurses to be well educated in the nuances of the patients' ECG findings and their associated physiologic responses promises to be high.

SUMMARY

The heart's electrical activity has been studied extensively throughout history, and evidence supporting the use of electrocardiography in clinical practice continues to evolve. The 12-lead ECG is an important noninvasive, objective diagnostic tool and indicator of cardiac function and continuous in-hospital cardiac monitoring provides evidence of patients' changing physiologic status. Understanding the normal ECG findings can help ensure safe, appropriate care of critically ill patients.

REFERENCES

1. Mehta NJ, Khan IA. Cardiology's 10 greatest discoveries of the 20th century. Tex Heart Inst J 2002;29(3):164–71.
2. Drew BJ, Califf RM, Funk M, et al. Practice standards for electrocardiographic monitoring in hospital settings: an American Heart Association Scientific Statement From the Councils on Cardiovascular Nursing, Clinical Cardiology, and Cardiovascular Disease in the Young: endorsed by the International Society of Computerized Electrocardiology and the American Association of Critical-Care Nurses. Circulation 2004;110(17):2721–46.
3. Drew B. Cardiac rhythm responses. 1. An important phenomenon for nursing practice, science, and research. Heart Lung 1989;18(1):8–16.
4. Goble AJ, Sloman G, Robinson JS. Mortality reduction in a coronary care unit. Br Med J 1966;1(5494):1005–9.
5. Fye WB. Resuscitating a circulation abstract to celebrate the 50th anniversary of the coronary care unit concept. Circulation 2011;124(17):1886–93.
6. Drew BJ. Celebrating the 100th birthday of the electrocardiogram: lessons learned from research in cardiac monitoring. Am J Crit Care 2002;11(4):378–86.
7. ECG Library. ECG timeline. A (not so) brief history of electrocardiography. 1996. 1786. Luigi Galvani. Available at: http://www.ecglibrary.com/ecghist.html. Accessed December 15, 2015.
8. ECG Library. ECG timeline. A (not so) brief history of electrocardiography 1996; 1865. Rudolph von Koelliker and Heinrich Muller. Available at: http://www.ecglibrary.com/ecghist.html. Accessed December 15, 2015.
9. Fye WB. Rudolf Albert von Koelliker. Clin Cardiol 1999;22(5):376–7.
10. Sykes AH. A D Waller and the electrocardiogram, 1887. Br Med J (Clin Res Ed) 1987;294(6584):1396–8.
11. Waller AD. A demonstration on man of electromotive changes accompanying the heart's beat. J Physiol 1887;8(5):229–34.

12. Drew BJ. Pitfalls and artifacts in electrocardiography. Cardiol Clin 2006;24(3): 309–15.
13. Adams MG, Drew BJ. Body position effects on the ECG: implication for ischemia monitoring. J Electrocardiol 1997;30(4):285–91.
14. Rivera-Ruiz M, Cajavilca C, Varon J. Einthoven's string galvanometer: the first electrocardiograph. Tex Heart Inst J 2008;35(2):174–8.
15. Einthoven W. Nobel lecture: the string galvanometer and the measurement of the action currents of the heart. 1925. Available at: http://www.nobelprize.org/nobel_prizes/medicine/laureates/1924/einthoven-lecture. Accessed December 9, 2015.
16. Van Mieghem C, Sabbe M, Knockaert D. The clinical value of the ECG in noncardiac conditions. Chest 2004;125(4):1561–76.
17. Kligfield P, Gettes LS, Bailey JJ, et al. Recommendations for the standardization and interpretation of the electrocardiogram: part i: the electrocardiogram and its technology a scientific statement from the American Heart Association Electrocardiography and Arrhythmias Committee, Council on Clinical Cardiology; the American College of Cardiology Foundation; and the Heart Rhythm Society endorsed by the International Society for Computerized Electrocardiology. J Am Coll Cardiol 2007;49(10):1109–27.
18. Sole M, Klein D, Moseley M. Dysrhythmia interpretation and management. Introduction to Critical Nursing, 6th edition. St Louis (MO): Elsevier; 2013. p. 98.
19. Yanowitz F. Introduction to ECG interpretation: The standard 12-lead ECG 2012; ECG Learning Center dedicated to Alan E. Lindsay. Available at: http://ecg.utah.edu/. Accessed May 11, 2016.
20. Katz A. Physiology of the heart. 4th edition. Philadelphia: Lippincott Williams & Wilkins; 2006.
21. Brubaker PH, Kitzman DW. Chronotropy: the Cinderella of heart failure pathophysiology and management. JACC Heart Fail 2013;1(3):267–9.
22. Goldberger AL. Introductory principles clinical electrocardiography: a simplified approach. 7th edition. Philadelphia: Mosby; 2006. p. 3–6.
23. Wiegand D. Cardiovascular system. In: Wiegand D, editor. AACN procedure manual for critical care. 6th edition. St Louis (MO): Elsevier Saunders; 2011. p. 415.
24. Nobelprize.org. The electrocardiogram, ECG. 2014. Available at: http://www.nobelprize.org/educational/medicine/ecg/ecg-readmore.htm. Accessed December 9, 2015.
25. Mason RE, Likar I. A new approach to stress tests in the diagnosis of myocardial ischemia. Trans Am Clin Climatol Assoc 1965;76:40–8.
26. Mason RE, Likar I. A new system of multiple-lead exercise electrocardiography. Am Heart J 1966;71(2):196–205.
27. Rijnbeek PR, van Herpen G, Bots ML, et al. Normal values of the electrocardiogram for ages 16–90 years. J Electrocardiol 2014;47(6):914–21.
28. Rautaharju PM, Surawicz B, Gettes LS. AHA/ACCF/HRS recommendations for the standardization and interpretation of the electrocardiogram: part IV: the ST segment, T and U waves, and the QT interval: a scientific statement from the American Heart Association Electrocardiography and Arrhythmias Committee, Council on Clinical Cardiology; the American College of Cardiology Foundation; and the Heart Rhythm Society: endorsed by the International Society for Computerized Electrocardiology. Circulation 2009;119(10):e241–50.
29. Surawicz BK, Knilans TK. Normal electrocardiogram: origin and description–chapter 1 - Chou's electrocardiography in clinical practice. 6th edition. Philadelphia: WB Saunders; 2008. p. 1–28.

30. Hasanien AA, Drew BJ, Howie-Esquivel J, et al. Prevalence and prognostic significance of long QT interval among patients with chest pain: selecting an optimum QT rate correction formula. J Electrocardiol 2013;46(4):336–42.
31. Hannibal GB. It started with Einthoven: the history of the ECG and cardiac monitoring. AACN Adv Crit Care 2011;22(1):93–6.
32. Alinier G, Gordon R, Harwood C, et al. 12-Lead ECG training: the way forward. Nurse Educ Today 2006;26(1):87–92.
33. Lejay A, Fang F, John R, et al. Ischemia reperfusion injury, ischemic conditioning and diabetes mellitus. J Mol Cell Cardiol 2016;91:11–22.
34. Hochstadt A, Meroz Y, Landesberg G. Myocardial dysfunction in severe sepsis and septic shock: more questions than answers? J Cardiothorac Vasc Anesth 2011;25(3):526–35.
35. Chatila W, Ani S, Guaglianone D, et al. Cardiac ischemia during weaning from mechanical ventilation. Chest 1996;109(6):1577–83.
36. Holanda M, Domínguez MJ, López-Espadas F, et al. Cardiac contusion following blunt chest trauma. Eur J Emerg Med 2006;13(6):373–6.
37. Fry AC, Farrington K. Management of acute renal failure. Postgrad Med J 2006; 82(964):106–16.
38. Moss AJ, Wojciech Zareba C, Benhorin J, et al. ISHNE guidelines for electrocardiographic evaluation of drug-related QT prolongation and other alterations in ventricular repolarization: task force summary. Ann Noninvasive Electrocardiol 2001;6(4):333–41.
39. Drew B, Harris P, Zègre-Hemsey J, et al. Insights into the problem of alarm fatigue with physiologic monitor devices: a comprehensive observational study of consecutive intensive care unit patients. PLoS One 2014;9(10):e110274.
40. Rautaharju PM. Eyewitness to history: landmarks in the development of computerized electrocardiography. J Electrocardiol 2015;49(1):1–6.
41. Salas-Boni R, Bai Y, Harris PRE, et al. False ventricular tachycardia alarm suppression in the ICU based on the discrete wavelet transform in the ECG signal. J Electrocardiol 2014;47(6):775–80.
42. de Bie J, Mortara DW, Clark TF. The development and validation of an early warning system to prevent the acquisition of 12-lead resting ECGs with interchanged electrode positions. J Electrocardiol 2014;47(6):794–7.
43. Bai Y, Do DH, Harris PRE, et al. Integrating monitor alarms with laboratory test results to enhance patient deterioration prediction. J Biomed Inform 2015;53: 81–92.
44. Quan D, Yong B, Adelita T, et al. Developing new predictive alarms based on ECG metrics for bradyasystolic cardiac arrest. Physiol Meas 2015;36(12):2405.
45. Macfarlane PW, Katibi IA, Hamde ST, et al. Racial differences in the ECG — selected aspects. J Electrocardiol 2014;47(6):809–14.
46. Pickham D, Flowers E, Drew BJ. Hyperglycemia is associated with QTC prolongation and mortality in the acutely ill. J Cardiovasc Nurs 2014;29(3):264–70.
47. Harris PRE, Stein PK, Fung GL, et al. Heart rate variability measured early in patients with evolving acute coronary syndrome and 1-year outcomes of rehospitalization and mortality. Vasc Health Risk Manag 2014;10:451–64.
48. Abtahi F, Snäll J, Aslamy B, et al. Biosignal PI, an affordable open-source ECG and respiration measurement system. Sensors (Basel) 2015;15(1):93–109.
49. Hsieh JC, Li AH, Yang CC. Mobile, cloud, and big data computing: contributions, challenges, and new directions in telecardiology. Int J Environ Res Public Health 2013;10(11):6131–53.

Bradyarrhythmias

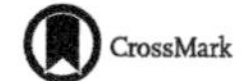

Clinical Presentation, Diagnosis, and Management

Shu-Fen Wung, PhD, RN, ACNP-BC

KEYWORDS

- Bradyarrhythmia • Sinus node dysfunction • Atrioventricular block
- Tachycardia-bradycardia syndrome • Sinus arrest

KEY POINTS

- Bradyarrhythmias can reflect normal physiologic responses, like sleeping, or reveal a number of rhythm disorders, including sinus node dysfunction and atrioventricular conduction disturbances.
- In patients with confirmed or suspected bradycardia, a thorough history and physical examination includes signs/symptoms, precipitating factors, medications, history of coronary artery disease, cardiac arrhythmia, and sudden death.
- Management is based on the severity of symptoms, underlying causes, presence of potentially reversible causes, presence of adverse signs, and risk of progression to asystole.

INTRODUCTION

Bradycardia, also known as bradyarrhythmia, is a common finding for both healthy individuals and those who are ill. This paper provides an overview on types and causes of bradyarrhythmia, the clinical presentation, diagnosis, and management.

DEFINITION OF BRADYCARDIA

In adults, bradycardia has traditionally been defined by consensus as a slow heart rate (HR) of fewer than 60 beats per minute (bpm).[1] This easily remembered HR threshold of 60 bpm for bradycardia has been challenged because it overdiagnoses bradycardia and is not consistent with published age- and sex-specific norms.[2–4] However, resting HR among the healthy, asymptomatic population varied greatly. A slow HR may be normal physiologically for some individuals, but may be inadequate for others. Classic work from Jose and Collison[5] (1970) showed that HR decreases with age. There is also

Disclosure Statement: The author has nothing to disclose.
Biobehavioral Health Science Division, The University of Arizona College of Nursing, 1305 North Martin Avenue, Tucson, AZ 85721-0203, USA
E-mail address: wung@arizona.edu

Crit Care Nurs Clin N Am 28 (2016) 297–308
http://dx.doi.org/10.1016/j.cnc.2016.04.003 ccnursing.theclinics.com
0899-5885/16/$ – see front matter © 2016 Elsevier Inc. All rights reserved.

a circadian cycle of HR, with fastest rates occurring between 1400 and 1700 hours and the slowest rates occurring between 0400 and 0600 hours.[6] During sleep, HR decreases by an average of 24 bpm in young adults[7,8] and by 14 bpm in those greater than 80 years of age.[6] Women have faster HR than men during both waking and sleeping periods, by an average of 10 bpm in young adults.[7,8] Spodick[9] reported that the "normal" range of HRs in the afternoon was 46 to 93 bpm for men and 51 to 95 bpm for women; thus, they proposed an HR of 50 bpm to be an appropriate level for defining bradycardia in adults.[9–11]

BRIEF OVERVIEW OF THE SINOATRIAL NODAL CONDUCTION SYSTEM

Cardiac rhythm is initiated and controlled by the sinoatrial (SA) node, the primary pacemaker of the heart. Current scientific knowledge indicates that the SA node structure consists of clusters of specialized cardiomyocytes enmeshed within strands of connective tissue or fibrosis.[12] In addition, there are also distinct SA conduction pathways that electrically connect the SA node to the right atrium. These SA conduction pathways play an important role in regulating the SA node automaticity and, thus, the maintenance of the HR.[12] Autonomic stimulation, ischemia, and/or structural remodeling can compromise the SA node pacemaker function and inhibit the impulse through the SA nodal conduction pathways (exit block).[12] The SA node exit block allows the impulse to originate from subsidiary pacemakers, such as the atrioventricular (AV) node and the specialized ventricular conduction system.

The HR is modulated by several factors, including the autonomic nervous system (the dynamic balance between sympathetic and parasympathetic nervous systems), the baroreceptors, the Bainbridge reflex, and the intrinsic HR.[13] The autonomic nervous system is reported to be more densely innervated in the cardiac conduction system than in the myocardium in other parts of the heart, with the SA node being the most densely innervated region of the conduction system.[14] This observation supports the central role of the autonomic nervous system in initiating and regulating the cardiac impulse. Sympathetic and parasympathetic nervous systems interact with adrenergic (α- and β-) and muscarinic receptors. In general, stimulation of β-adrenoceptors increases HR, whereas stimulation of muscarinic receptors decreases HR.[15]

The idea that the cardiac impulse originates from a very focal region in the SA node has been challenged. Boineau and associates[16] demonstrated that humans have a widely distributed physiologic pacemaker complex extending across a significantly larger area of atrial tissue. The concept of an "atrial pacemaker complex," including the SA node, SA nodal conduction pathways, and the surrounding atrial myocardium, is proposed to initiate normal atrial or sinus rhythm.[16]

TYPES OF BRADYARRHYTHMIAS

Bradyarrhythmias can reflect normal physiologic responses, as in sleeping, or reveal a number of rhythm disorders, including sinus node dysfunction and AV conduction disturbances.[17] Sinus node dysfunction is caused by a depressed automaticity or an impaired SA node and atrial impulse formation and/or propagation. Sinus node dysfunction, sometimes used interchangeably with "sick sinus syndrome,"[18,19] refers to a spectrum of heart rhythm disturbances, including sinus bradycardia (**Fig. 1**), sinus arrest, sinus exit block, and tachycardia–bradycardia syndrome.[18] Of note, the bedside monitor is sensitive to artifactual noise in the electrocardiogram (ECG) signal so that artifact can generate a false-positive bardycardiac alarm (**Fig. 2**). Chronotropic incompetence, defined as the inadequate HR response to increased activity or

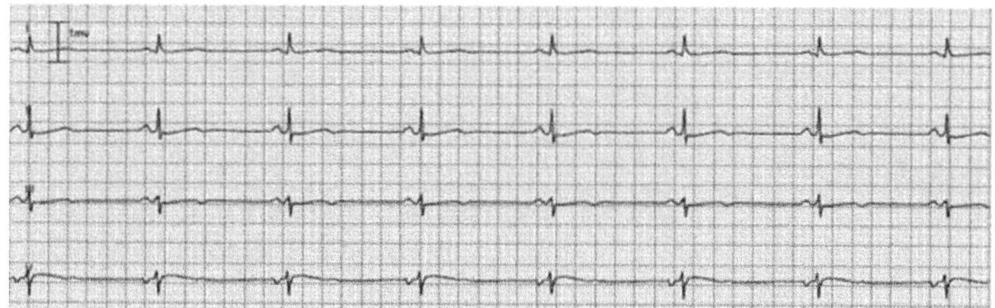

Fig. 1. Sinus bradycardia. Sinus bradycardia is bradycardia in the presence of normal sinus rhythm. The P wave is normally positive in leads I, II, and III and biphasic in lead V_1. The PR is normal at less than 0.2 second. The QRS is narrow. Because there are 34 small boxes between regular R-R intervals, the heart rate calculation is 1500/34 = 44 beats per minute (bpm). (*Courtesy of* Shu-Fen Wung, PhD, RN, ACNP, FAAN, Tucson, AZ.)

demand, without identifiable causes, is also considered sinus node dysfunction (**Table 1**).[20]

AV conduction disturbances include first-, second-, high-, and third-degree (or complete) AV blocks. First-degree AV block is defined as a PR interval of greater than 0.2 seconds with a 1:1 AV conduction ratio on the ECG. There are 2 types of second-degree AV block: Mobitz types I and II, categorized by intermittently dropped ventricular beats. Mobitz type I block, also known as Wenckebach, is defined as a progressive increase in the PR interval until a P wave fails to conduct to the ventricle. Mobitz type II block is a periodic AV block with constant PR intervals in the conducted beats. Advanced or high-degree AV block consists of multiple P waves that are blocked, but without third-degree AV block present. Third-degree AV block occurs when atrial and ventricular activities are independent of each other (AV dissociation) and AV conduction is absent. Bradycardia is often associated with second-degree or third-degree AV block.

CAUSES OF BRADYARRHYTHMIAS

Multiple physiologic and pathophysiological causes can produce bradyarrhythmias (**Box 1**). A selected discussion of these factors is summarized herein.

Athletes

In endurance athletes, sinus bradycardia with an HR of less than 40 bpm is common and sinus pauses lasting more than 2 seconds were found in 37% of athletes during

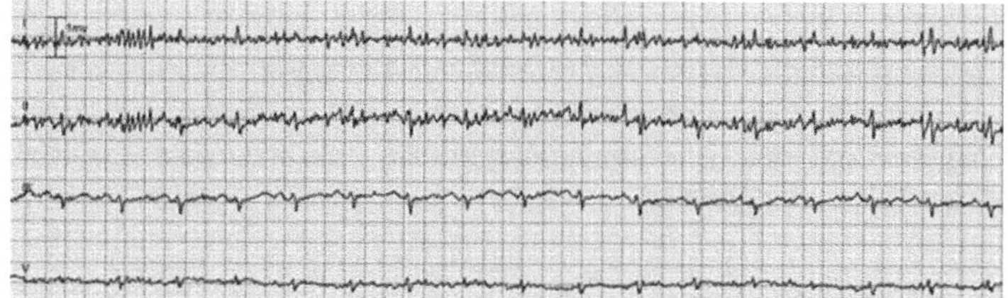

Fig. 2. False Interpretation of bradycardia. This is a false-positive bradycardia alarm owing to low-amplitude QRS complexes and artifact interfering with the computer algorithm. The monitor reports a heart rate (HR) of 56 beats per minute (bpm), but there are 15 small boxes between the regular R-R interval; thus, the correct HR should be 1500/15 = 100 bpm. This demonstrates that a clinician's visual interpretation of cardiac rate is important in the determination of bradyarrhythmias. (*Courtesy of* Shu-Fen Wung, PhD, RN, ACNP, FAAN, Tucson, AZ.)

Table 1
Types of bradyarrhythmias

Type	Definition
Sinus node dysfunction	
Sinus arrest	A pause in the sinus rhythm owing to failure of the sinus node to depolarize (impulse formation).
Sinus exit block	A pause owing to conduction failure from the sinus node to the surrounding atrium. The duration of this pause is a multiple of the sinus P-P interval.
Sinus bradycardia	Bradycardia in conjunction with normal sinus rhythm owing to depressed automaticity of the sinus node.
Tachycardia-bradycardia syndrome	A combination of tachycardia (atrial fibrillation, atrial flutter, etc) and sinus bradycardia, also called sick sinus syndrome.
Chronotropic incompetence	Inadequate heart rate response to increased activity or demand, without identifiable causes.
AV conduction disturbances	
First-degree AV block	A PR interval of >0.2 s with a 1:1 AV conduction ratio.
Second-degree AV block	Categorized by intermittently dropped ventricular beat.
Mobitz type I (Wenckebach)	A progressive increase in the PR interval until a P wave fails to conduct to the ventricle.
Mobitz type II	Periodic AV block with constant PR intervals in the conducted beats.
Advanced or high-degree AV block	Multiple P waves that are blocked but without third-degree AV block present.
Third-degree AV block with junctional or ventricular escape rhythm	Complete dissociation of atrial and ventricular electrical conduction, thus, none of the signals generated above the AV node are conducted to the ventricles; thus, junctional or ventricular escape rhythms are approximately 30–50 beats per minute.

Abbreviation: AV, atrioventricular.

sleep.[21] Recent research has shown that the type of sport influences the level and mechanisms of resting bradycardia.[22] For example, resting bradycardia in runners depends on higher vagal tone, whereas resting bradycardia in cyclists is probably associated with cardiac hypertrophy.

Aging

An explanation for the slower HR as an individual grows older is the sympathetic dominance of the cardiac conduction system in infancy and gradual transition into a sympathetic and parasympathetic codominance in adulthood.[23] Sinus node dysfunction is primarily a disease of the elderly. Recent work has shown that an age-induced increase of SA node fibrosis is correlated strongly with slowed intrinsic HR and slowed SA node conduction.[24]

Box 1
Causes of bradyarrhythmias

- Athlete
- Aging
- Medications effects/overdoses
  - β-Blockers, including eye drops for glaucoma (timolol)
  - Calcium channel blockers, nondihydropyridine
  - Antiarrhythmics (class I and III)
  - Digoxin
  - Other sympatholytic antihypertensive (clonidine, prazosin, etc)
  - Other (guanfacine extended release, corticosteroid, donepezil, narcotics, anesthetics, fingolimod, thiopentone sodium, etc)
- Genetics
- Acute myocardial ischemia/infarction (right and/or circumflex artery)
- Seizure
- Other conditions
  - Myocarditis
  - Infection and febrile illness (encephalitis, dengue hemorrhagic fever, etc)
  - Endocrine (hypothyroidism, hypogonadotropic hypogonadism, etc)
  - Anorexia nervosa
  - Hypothermia, hypoglycemia
  - Electrolyte disturbances (eg, hyperkalemia, hypokalemia, hypocalcemia)
  - Diving
  - Infiltrative disorders
  - Collagen vascular diseases
  - Conduction system injuries (eg, surgery)
  - Altered autonomic influence (eg, nausea/vomiting, neurally mediated syncope [vasovagal syncope])
  - Systemic hypoxia
  - Sleep apnea

Medications

A number of pharmacologic agents, such as β-adrenergic blockers (metoprolol, nebivolol, etc), nondihydropyridine calcium channel blockers (diltiazem, verapamil, etc), antiarrhythmics, digoxin, and other sympathomimetic antihypertensives (clonidine, prazosin, etc) are known to cause bradycardia. Importantly, topical ophthalmic medications, such as timolol maleate, used for treatment of glaucoma and ocular hypertension, are absorbed from the eye into the systemic circulation and can causes systemic adrenergic β-blocking, leading to AV block and bradycardia.[25] Bradycardia has also been reported with other noncardiovascular pharmacologic agents in standard doses or overdoses. These include but are not limited to guanfacine extended release, corticosteroid, donepezil, narcotics, and anesthetics.

Genetics

There is a genetic component of bradyarrhythmias.[26] For example, familiar forms of primary sinus bradycardia have been associated with several genetic mutations, including the hyperpolarization-activated cyclic nucleotide–gated potassium channel 4 (*HCN4*) gene, the sodium channel voltage gated type V alpha subunit (*SCN5A*) gene, and the ankyrin 2, neuronal (*ANK2*) gene.[27] Genes affecting enzymes involved in medication metabolism and elimination can also contribute to bradyarrhythmias. For example, cytochrome P450 family 2 subfamily D polypeptide 6 (CYP2D6) is the main enzyme contributing to the metabolism of several β-blockers. Several genetic polymorphisms of the *CYP2D6* gene, such as CYP2D6 *4/*4, lead to no enzyme activity. Patients with these genetic defects, also called poor metabolizers of CYP2D6, are at increased risk of bradycardia.[28]

Acute Myocardial Ischemia of Infarction

Bradyarrhythmias can be owing to myocardial ischemia or infarction involving the proximal right and/or circumflex artery or the coronary artery supplying blood flow to the sinus node or to the AV node.

Seizures

Ictal bradycardia and asystole have been reported in 2% to 37% and in 1% to 16% of seizures, respectively.[29] The mechanism for seizure-related bradyarrhythmia is unclear. Because ictal bradyarrhythmias are preceded frequently by transitory tachycardia, the current thinking suggests that bradyarrhythmias may involve a reflex to counteract tachycardia by excessive activation of the vagal nerve.[29]

Gender

Based on a large pacemaker implantation registry in Germany involving 17,826 patients, it was reported that women are more likely to have sick sinus syndrome but less likely to have AV block as a primary pacemaker indication.[30] The underlying mechanisms for these gender differences are unknown and require further investigation.

Other Conditions

Other conditions that result in bradyarrhythmia may include infection or febrile illnesses (encephalitis, dengue hemorrhagic fever, etc), endocrinologic abnormalities (hypothyroidism), anorexia nervosa, hypothermia, hypoglycemia, electrolyte disturbances (eg, hyperkalemia), infiltrative disease, collagen vascular disease, trauma to the cardiac conduction system, hypoxia, and other complications.[31]

CLINICAL PRESENTATION

Cardiac output is determined by the left ventricular stroke volume multiplied by the HR. Patients with bradycardia may be asymptomatic if changes in stroke volume compensate for the decrease in HR. Symptoms of bradycardia can be diverse and related to reduce cardiac output, resulting in the hypoperfusion of vital organs. The symptoms can be nonspecific and chronic, including dyspnea on exertion, exercise intolerance, fatigue, and weakness. However, symptoms may be severe including syncope, lightheadedness or dizziness, palpitation, angina, or a change of mental status.[17,32]

EVALUATION AND DIAGNOSIS OF BRADYARRHYTHMIAS

In asymptomatic individuals, bradycardia may be noted as an incidental finding during a routine checkup or on an ECG obtained for other purposes. In patients with confirmed or suspected bradycardia, a thorough history and physical examination should include documentation of associated signs and symptoms of hypoperfusion and precipitating factors, medications (including nasal and ophthalmic routes), personal and family history (coronary artery disease, cardiac arrhythmia, and sudden death), and possible causes of SA node dysfunction or AV block (see **Box 1**).

Diagnostic Testing

Basic laboratory studies should include tests of electrolytes, glucose, toxicology screening for narcotics and digitalis level (if the patient is on digoxin), and thyroid function. To establish the diagnosis of bradyarrhythmia, it is crucial to find a causal relationship between patient symptoms and abnormalities on the ECG.[33] A standard 12-lead ECG is used to determine the presence and type of bradyarrhythmia and/or the presence of structural cardiac disease, such as prior or acute myocardial ischemia/infarction. Because bradyarrhythmia may be intermittent, prolonged cardiac monitoring should be considered if a 12-lead ECG does not yield a diagnosis. Selection of these modalities is based on symptom severity and frequency. A 24- to 48-hour Holter monitor is generally the first-line choice in patients with frequent symptoms. If suspicion of arrhythmia is high, but the Holter monitoring is nondiagnostic and the patient is experiencing intermittent symptoms, longer cardiac monitoring of 1 to 4 weeks using noninvasive mobile cardiovascular telemetry or event monitoring is the next step. Implantable loop recorders are available to provide continuous cardiac monitoring from any number of months to 3 years. These ambulatory cardiac monitoring devices and costs have been summarized.[34] In addition, invasive electrophysiologic studies may be used to evaluate sinus node dysfunction and AV blocks in patients with known or suspected bradyarrhythmias. For example, electrophysiologic studies are appropriate when sinus node dysfunction is suspected in symptomatic patients. During electrophysiologic studies, AV nodal and His–Purkinje conduction durations are precisely measured on a His-bundle ECG so the site of the block is identified, but a causal relation between an arrhythmia and symptoms has not been established.[35]

Chronotropic incompetence can be diagnosed by an incremental dynamic exercise testing when the HR fails to reach an arbitrary percentage (≥80%) of the age-predicted maximal HR (usually 220 – age).[36] Tilt-table testing may be used to diagnose neurally mediated syncope (or vasovagal syncope) by eliciting syncopal symptoms during provocation of neurally mediated hypotension and/or bradycardia.[37]

MANAGEMENT

Management of bradycardia is based on the severity of symptoms, underlying causes, presence of potentially reversible causes, presence of adverse signs (**Table 2**), and risk of progression to asystole (**Box 2**).[38] Some bradycardia may not require treatment or may involve correction of reversible causes for bradycardia. For example, bradycardia develops in patients with obstructive sleep apnea and hypoxia; appropriately treated sleep apnea may eliminate bradycardia. When a patient is unstable

Table 2
Adverse signs indicating unstable condition related to arrhythmia

Adverse Signs	Signs and Symptoms of Instability
Shock	Pallor, sweating, cold and clammy extremities, impaired consciousness, hypotension (systolic blood pressure <90 mm Hg)
Syncope	Loss of consciousness
Heart failure	Pulmonary edema, hepatic engorgement
Myocardial ischemia	Angina, acute ischemia on electrocardiogram

Data from Soar J, Nolan JP, Bottiger BW, et al. European Resuscitation Council Guidelines for Resuscitation 2015: Section 3. Adult advanced life support. Resuscitation 2015;95:100–47.

Box 2
High risk of progression to asystole

- Recent asystole
- Mobitz type II AV block
- Complete AV block with wide QRS
- Ventricular pause greater than 3 seconds

Abbreviation: AV, atrioventricular.
Data from Soar J, Nolan JP, Bottiger BW, et al. European Resuscitation Council Guidelines for Resuscitation 2015: Section 3. Adult advanced life support. Resuscitation 2015;95:100–47.

(see **Table 2**), it is important to determine the cause of the patient's instability to direct treatment properly. For example, if a patient becomes hypotensive and develops a bradycardia owing to respiratory failure and severe hypoxemia, treating the bradycardia without treating the hypoxemia is unlikely to improve the patient's instability. When adverse signs or a high risk of progression to asystole are evident, immediate treatment for bradycardia should be initiated.[39] Patient assessment using a rapid evaluation tool such as the Airway, Breathing, Circulation, Disability, Exposure (ABCDE) approach is recommended for acute unstable bradycardia (see **Table 2**).[39]

Pharmacologic Therapy

Initial treatments are pharmacologic, with pacing being reserved for patients unresponsive to pharmacologic treatments or with risk factors for asystole (see **Box 2**).

Atropine sulfate

If bradycardia produces acute signs and symptoms of instability (see **Table 2**), the first-line treatment is atropine sulfate.[40] Atropine is an antimuscarinic medication that reverses cholinergic-mediated decreases in HR and AV conduction. Atropine improves HR and the signs and symptoms associated with bradycardia.[40] The recommended initial atropine dose for bradycardia in adults is 0.5 mg intravenously, repeated if necessary every 3 to 5 minutes to a maximum total dose of 3 mg.[40] It is important to provide adequate doses of atropine because doses of less than 0.5 mg may result in paradoxic further slowing of the HR.[41] For adult patients who are morbidly obese, the dose of atropine should be calculated using lean body weight.[42] Atropine should be considered a temporary measure and should not delay implementation of a pacemaker for patients with symptomatic and/or unstable bradyarrhythmia or sinus arrest. Atropine should be used cautiously in patients with acute coronary syndrome; an increased HR may worsen acute ischemia or infarction.[41]

Alternative medications

Intravenous infusion of β-adrenergic agonists with HR accelerating effects (eg, dopamine, epinephrine, isoproterenol) can be effective if the bradycardia is unresponsive to atropine.[40] Results from various studies[43,44] have showed paradoxic slowing of the HR, AV block, and sinus arrest when atropine was administered to patients after cardiac transplantation. In these patients, β-adrenergic agonists as treatment measures are preferred over atropine.[40] For patients with Mobitz type II or third-degree AV blocks with a wide QRS complex, the location of a block is likely below the AV node; thus, the patient is unlikely to be responsive to atropine or β-adrenergic agonists. Alternative medications, such as glucagon, may also be appropriate in special circumstances if β-blocker or calcium channel blocker overdose is suspected.[41]

Cardiac Pacing

Temporary pacing

Temporary pacing should be initiated immediately in patients suffering from severe or clinically significant episodes of bradyarrhythmia and asystole,[45] if there is no response to atropine or if atropine is unlikely to be effective. It is an emergency measure to provide temporary ventricular rate support, and thus cardiac output, for adequate perfusion of the vital organs until permanent pacing can be arranged. There are several forms of temporary pacing: transcutaneous, esophageal, epicardial, or percutaneous transvenous. Transcutaneous pacing is done by applying adhesive pads to the chest in anteroposterior or anteroapical configuration. Esophageal pacing is rarely used. Traditionally, transvenous pacing is used to stabilize patients suffering from hemodynamic unstable bradyarrhythmia. This procedure is painful in conscious patients, and therefore requires sedatives or anesthetics. Indications for pacemaker use and strategies to manipulate temporary pacemakers to optimize hemodynamics are of utmost importance.[45]

Permanent pacing

Permanent pacemaker implantation is the only effective treatment for symptomatic bradycardia[20] (**Fig. 3**). The decision regarding the need for a pacemaker is influenced by the presence of symptoms directly attributable to bradycardia. For adults with SA node dysfunction, indications for permanent pacemaker implantation include frequent symptomatic sinus pauses, symptomatic chronotropic incompetence, and symptomatic sinus bradycardia that result from required drug therapy for medical conditions.[20] Recommendations for permanent pacemaker implantation for second-degree and

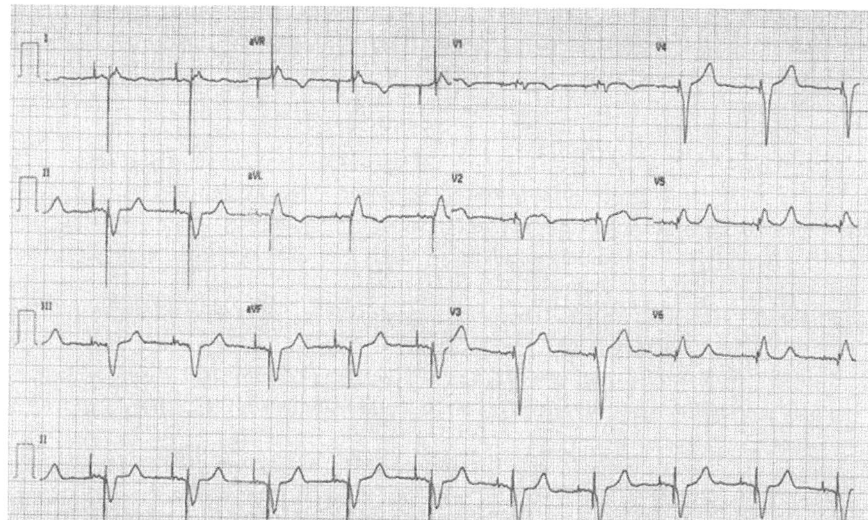

Fig. 3. An example of a dual-chambered pacemaker. This is a standard 12-lead electrocardiogram recorded in a 79-year-old man with a dual-chamber pacemaker. The bottom tracing lead II is the simultaneous recording of rhythms above. In dual-chamber pacemakers, electrodes are inserted into both the right atrium and right ventricle. Atrial and ventricular pacemaker spikes are seen before each P wave and QRS, respectively, at a rate of 60 beats per minute. There is a programmable atrioventricular delay, interval between the atrial and ventricular pacemaker spikes, similar to PR interval seen in physiologic conduction. (*Courtesy of* Shu-Fen Wung, PhD, RN, ACNP, FAAN, Tucson, AZ.)

third-degree AV block have also been summarized in the American College of Cardiology and American Heart Association guidelines.[20] In general, asymptomatic episodes of sinus bradycardia (with the HR as low as 40 bpm), sinus pauses of up to 3 seconds, and first-degree and Mobitz type I AV block are not considered to be indications for permanent pacemaker implantation. It is crucial for clinicians to distinguish between physiologic bradycardia owing to autonomic conditions or athletic training effects and inappropriate bradycardia that requires permanent cardiac pacing. For example, in trained athletes, sinus bradycardia does not require permanent pacemaker implantation. Pacemaker placement is not necessary in patients with anorexia nervosa because reversal of cardiac conduction disturbances occur with proper nutrition and weight normalization.[46]

SUMMARY

Bradyarrhythmias are common clinical findings and they consist of various physiologic and pathologic conditions (sinus node dysfunction and AV conduction disturbances). Bradyarrhythmias can be benign, requiring no treatment; however, acute unstable bradycardia can lead to cardiac arrest. In patients with confirmed or suspected bradycardia, a thorough history and physical examination should include possible causes of SA node dysfunction or AV block. Management of bradycardia is based on the severity of symptoms, the underlying causes, the presence of potentially reversible causes, the presence of adverse signs, and the risk of progression to asystole. Pharmacologic therapy and/or pacing are used to manage unstable or symptomatic bradyarrhythmias.[40]

REFERENCES

1. Kossmann CE. The normal electrocardiogram. Circulation 1953;8(6):920–36.
2. Mason JW, Ramseth DJ, Chanter DO, et al. Electrocardiographic reference ranges derived from 79,743 ambulatory subjects. J Electrocardiol 2007;40(3): 228–34.
3. Macfarlane PW, Lawrie TDV. Comprehensive electrocardiology: theory and practice in health and disease. New York: Pergamon Press; 1989.
4. Ostchega Y, Porter KS, Hughes J, et al. Resting pulse rate reference data for children, adolescents, and adults: United States, 1999-2008. Natl Health Stat Rep 2011;(41):1–16.
5. Jose AD, Collison D. The normal range and determinants of the intrinsic heart rate in man. Cardiovasc Res 1970;4(2):160–7.
6. Kantelip JP, Sage E, Duchene-Marullaz P. Findings on ambulatory electrocardiographic monitoring in subjects older than 80 years. Am J Cardiol 1986;57(6): 398–401.
7. Brodsky M, Wu D, Denes P, et al. Arrhythmias documented by 24 hour continuous electrocardiographic monitoring in 50 male medical students without apparent heart disease. Am J Cardiol 1977;39(3):390–5.
8. Sobotka PA, Mayer JH, Bauernfeind RA, et al. Arrhythmias documented by 24-hour continuous ambulatory electrocardiographic monitoring in young women without apparent heart disease. Am Heart J 1981;101(6):753–9.
9. Spodick DH. Normal sinus heart rate: appropriate rate thresholds for sinus tachycardia and bradycardia. South Med J 1996;89(7):666–7.
10. Spodick DH, Raju P, Bishop RL, et al. Operational definition of normal sinus heart rate. Am J Cardiol 1992;69(14):1245–6.

11. Kozik TM, Wung SF. Acquired long QT syndrome: frequency, onset, and risk factors in intensive care patients. Crit Care Nurse 2012;32(5):32–41.
12. Fedorov VV, Glukhov AV, Chang R. Conduction barriers and pathways of the sinoatrial pacemaker complex: their role in normal rhythm and atrial arrhythmias. Am J Physiol Heart Circ Physiol 2012;302(9):H1773–83.
13. Camm AJ, Fei L. Chronotropic incompetence–Part I: normal regulation of the heart rate. Clin Cardiol 1996;19(5):424–8.
14. Crick SJ, Wharton J, Sheppard MN, et al. Innervation of the human cardiac conduction system. A quantitative immunohistochemical and histochemical study. Circulation 1994;89(4):1697–708.
15. Brodde OE, Bruck H, Leineweber K, et al. Presence, distribution and physiological function of adrenergic and muscarinic receptor subtypes in the human heart. Basic Res Cardiol 2001;96(6):528–38.
16. Boineau JP, Canavan TE, Schuessler RB, et al. Demonstration of a widely distributed atrial pacemaker complex in the human heart. Circulation 1988;77(6):1221–37.
17. Dresing TJ, L Wilkoff B. Bradyarrhythmias. Curr Treat Options Cardiovasc Med 2001;3(4):291–8.
18. Ferrer MI. The sick sinus syndrome in atrial disease. JAMA 1968;206(3):645–6.
19. Bashour TT. Classification of sinus node dysfunction. Am Heart J 1985;110(6):1251–6.
20. Epstein AE, DiMarco JP, Ellenbogen KA, et al. 2012 ACCF/AHA/HRS focused update incorporated into the ACCF/AHA/HRS 2008 guidelines for device-based therapy of cardiac rhythm abnormalities: a report of the American College of Cardiology Foundation/American Heart Association Task Force on Practice Guidelines and the Heart Rhythm Society. J Am Coll Cardiol 2013;61(3):e6–75.
21. Viitasalo MT, Kala R, Eisalo A. Ambulatory electrocardiographic recording in endurance athletes. Br Heart J 1982;47(3):213–20.
22. Azevedo LF, Perlingeiro PS, Hachul DT, et al. Sport modality affects bradycardia level and its mechanisms of control in professional athletes. Int J Sports Med 2014;35(11):954–9.
23. Chow LT, Chow SS, Anderson RH, et al. Autonomic innervation of the human cardiac conduction system: changes from infancy to senility–an immunohistochemical and histochemical analysis. Anat Rec 2001;264(2):169–82.
24. Akoum N, McGann C, Vergara G, et al. Atrial fibrosis quantified using late gadolinium enhancement MRI is associated with sinus node dysfunction requiring pacemaker implant. J Cardiovasc Electrophysiol 2012;23(1):44–50.
25. Nieminen T, Lehtimaki T, Maenpaa J, et al. Ophthalmic timolol: plasma concentration and systemic cardiopulmonary effects. Scand J Clin Lab Invest 2007;67(2):237–45.
26. Wung SF, Hickey KT, Taylor JY, et al. Cardiovascular genomics. J Nurs Scholarsh 2013;45(1):60–8.
27. Milano A, Vermeer AM, Lodder EM, et al. HCN4 mutations in multiple families with bradycardia and left ventricular noncompaction cardiomyopathy. J Am Coll Cardiol 2014;64(8):745–56.
28. Bijl MJ, Visser LE, van Schaik RH, et al. Genetic variation in the CYP2D6 gene is associated with a lower heart rate and blood pressure in beta-blocker users. Clin Pharmacol Ther 2009;85(1):45–50.
29. Duplyakov D, Golovina G, Lyukshina N, et al. Syncope, seizure-induced bradycardia and asystole: two cases and review of clinical and pathophysiological features. Seizure 2014;23(7):506–11.

30. Nowak B, Misselwitz B, Expert committee 'Pacemaker', et al. Do gender differences exist in pacemaker implantation?–results of an obligatory external quality control program. Europace 2010;12(2):210–5.
31. Swift J. Assessment and treatment of patients with acute unstable bradycardia. Nurs Stand 2013;27(22):48–56 [quiz: 58].
32. Rubenstein JJ, Schulman CL, Yurchak PM, et al. Clinical spectrum of the sick sinus syndrome. Circulation 1972;46(1):5–13.
33. Wung SF, Kozik T. Electrocardiographic evaluation of cardiovascular status. J Cardiovasc Nurs 2008;23(2):169–74.
34. Semelka M, Gera J, Usman S. Sick sinus syndrome: a review. Am Fam Physician 2013;87(10):691–6.
35. Zipes DP, DiMarco JP, Gillette PC, et al. Guidelines for clinical intracardiac electrophysiological and catheter ablation procedures. A report of the American College of Cardiology/American Heart Association Task Force on Practice Guidelines (Committee on Clinical Intracardiac Electrophysiologic and Catheter Ablation Procedures), developed in collaboration with the North American Society of Pacing and Electrophysiology. J Am Coll Cardiol 1995;26(2):555–73.
36. Brubaker PH, Kitzman DW. Chronotropic incompetence: causes, consequences, and management. Circulation 2011;123(9):1010–20.
37. Benditt DG, Ferguson DW, Grubb BP, et al. Tilt table testing for assessing syncope. American College of Cardiology. J Am Coll Cardiol 1996;28(1):263–75.
38. Kozik TM, Wung SF. Cardiac arrest from acquired long QT syndrome: a case report. Heart Lung 2009;38(3):238–42.
39. Soar J, Nolan JP, Bottiger BW, et al. European Resuscitation Council Guidelines for Resuscitation 2015: section 3. Adult advanced life support. Resuscitation 2015;95:100–47.
40. Neumar RW, Otto CW, Link MS, et al. Part 8: adult advanced cardiovascular life support: 2010 American Heart Association Guidelines for Cardiopulmonary Resuscitation and Emergency Cardiovascular Care. Circulation 2010; 122(18 Suppl 3):S729–67.
41. Dauchot P, Gravenstein JS. Effects of atropine on the electrocardiogram in different age groups. Clin Pharmacol Ther 1971;12(2):274–80.
42. Carron M, Veronese S. Atropine sulfate for treatment of bradycardia in a patient with morbid obesity: what may happen when you least expect it. BMJ Case Rep 2015;2015:1–3.
43. Bernheim A, Fatio R, Kiowski W, et al. Atropine often results in complete atrioventricular block or sinus arrest after cardiac transplantation: an unpredictable and dose-independent phenomenon. Transplantation 2004;77(8):1181–5.
44. Brunner-La Rocca HP, Kiowski W, Bracht C, et al. Atrioventricular block after administration of atropine in patients following cardiac transplantation. Transplantation 1997;63(12):1838–9.
45. Sullivan BL, Bartels K, Hamilton N. Insertion and management of temporary pacemakers. Semin Cardiothorac Vasc Anesth 2016;20(1):52–62.
46. Mont L, Castro J, Herreros B, et al. Reversibility of cardiac abnormalities in adolescents with anorexia nervosa after weight recovery. J Am Acad Child Adolesc Psychiatry 2003;42(7):808–13.

Paroxysmal Supraventricular Tachycardia

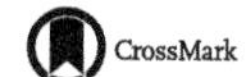

Pathophysiology, Diagnosis, and Management

Salah S. Al-Zaiti, RN, ANP-BC, PhD*, Kathy S. Magdic, RN, ACNP-BC, DNP

KEYWORDS

- Paroxysmal supraventricular tachycardia • Wolff-Parkinson-White syndrome
- Supraventricular arrhythmia • Accessory pathways

KEY POINTS

- Paroxysmal supraventricular tachycardia (PSVT) is a distinct clinical syndrome associated with intermittent episodes of palpitations of sudden onset and abrupt termination.
- The electrocardiogram pattern demonstrates regular tachycardia rhythm (150–240 bpm), narrow QRS complexes (<120 milliseconds), and hidden or inverted P waves.
- PSVT develops when separate pathways with different refractory and conduction speeds exist, resulting in atrioventricular nodal re-entry or re-entry through accessory or concealed pathways.
- Symptoms in almost all patients can be controlled or eliminated with appropriate therapy.
- In the absence of structural heart disease, catheter ablation can provide a long-term cure.

INTRODUCTION

During the normal cardiac cycle, the atria and the ventricles contract and relax in a synchronized fashion, manifested in normal sinus rhythm on the electrocardiogram (ECG). Physiologic demand (exercise, stress, and so on) results in appropriate acceleration of the heart rate[1]; however, a heart rate greater than 100 to 150 beats per minute (bpm) during rest, in the absence of appropriate physiologic response, might result in compromised cardiac output.[2] Patients might be completely asymptomatic, or feel isolated palpitations, complain about sudden chest pain, or even present with syncope if tachycardia is severe. Health care professionals frequently encounter patients with such symptomatic tachycardia; appropriate understanding

Disclosure Statement: The authors have nothing to disclose.

Department of Acute and Tertiary Care, School of Nursing, University of Pittsburgh, 3500 Victoria Street, 336 VB, Pittsburgh, PA 15261, USA
* Corresponding author.
E-mail address: ssa33@pitt.edu

Crit Care Nurs Clin N Am 28 (2016) 309–316
http://dx.doi.org/10.1016/j.cnc.2016.04.005 ccnursing.theclinics.com
0899-5885/16/$ – see front matter © 2016 Elsevier Inc. All rights reserved.

of pathophysiologic mechanisms underlying cardiac rhythms can guide proper diagnosis and management of these patients.

Case history

Dave, a 17-year-old healthy adolescent, experienced sudden-onset palpitations and lightheadedness while having dinner at home. The palpitations stopped abruptly when his parents splashed some water on his face. Because of a similar episode a week earlier, he was evaluated at the emergency department. His initial evaluation was normal as was his resting 12-lead ECG. He was referred to a cardiologist to discuss diagnosis and subsequent therapy.

DEFINITION AND PREVALENCE

Supraventricular tachycardia (SVT) is a general term used to describe any narrow (<120 milliseconds) QRS complex tachycardia (>100 bpm) suggestive of tissue involvement from or above the bundle of His. Paroxysmal supraventricular tachycardia (PSVT) is a distinct clinical subtype associated with regular tachycardia (150–240 bpm) of sudden onset and abrupt termination (paroxysmal).[3,4] Most patients have an unremarkable past medical history with no associated structural heart disease. The cause of the PSVT is frequently attributed to the re-entry mechanism.[5,6]

There are more than 500,000 patients with PSVT in the United States, with nearly 90,000 newly diagnosed cases every year. Most cases of PSVT are first diagnosed between the ages of 12 and 30 years of age. These patients usually present with abrupt onset of palpitations often associated with symptoms, including dizziness, syncope, chest pain, shortness of breath, weakness, and/or diaphoresis.[5] Approximately 5% of cases of PSVT are attributed to Wolff-Parkinson-White (WPW) syndrome.[6] Risk stratification is important given that those with WPW syndrome experience a significantly increased risk of sudden cardiac arrest compared with the general population.[7]

MECHANISM AND PATHOPHYSIOLOGY

In a normal heart, the electrical impulse originates at the sinoatrial (SA) node and travels in an anterograde direction to the ventricles through the atrioventricular (AV) node, which serves as a gatekeeper to maintain the synchrony of contractions between the atria and the ventricles (**Fig. 1**A).[8] This normal signal propagation depends on the electrical homogeneity of adjacent conducting pathways characterized by similar refractory and conduction periods. When there are 2 separate pathways with different refractory and conduction speeds, a re-entry circuit may develop.[6]

PSVT is caused by re-entry and is typically classified according to the anatomic location of the re-entry circuit. AV nodal re-entrant tachycardia (AVNRT) is the most common type of PSVT. It develops when 2 nondistinct, adjacent conduction pathways (α and β pathways) that lie within or near the AV node have different conduction velocities resulting in differences in conduction speeds and refractory periods. When an electrical impulse reaches these adjacent fibers, one fiber may be refractory and unable to conduct the impulse, potentially resulting in the impulse traveling through one pathway but not the other. When a critically timed premature atrial contraction travels anterograde through one pathway (α, or the "fast path") and then backward in a retrograde direction to its origin through the refractory pathway (β, or the "slow path"), a unidirectional circuit (re-entry) develops and triggers PSVT (**Fig. 1**B).[6,8–10] This re-entry circuit dominates the ECG signal so that the normal occurring SA node activity

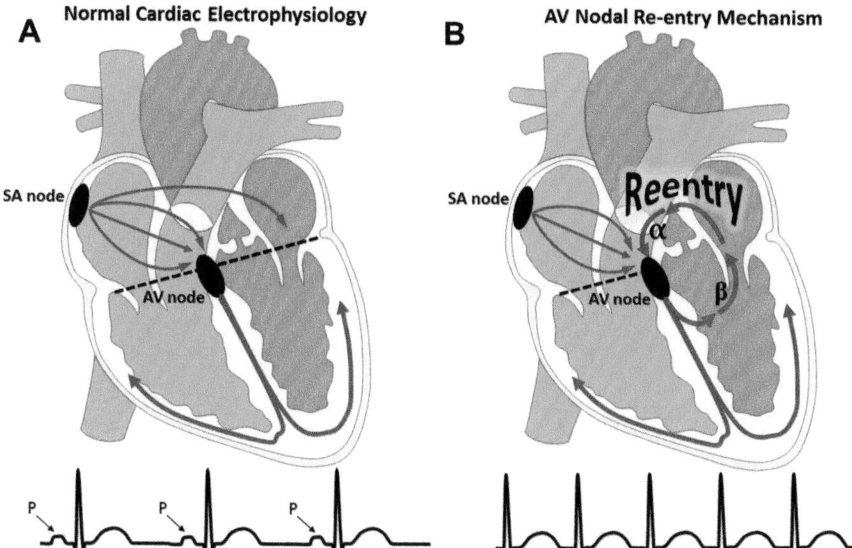

Fig. 1. Common PSVT mechanisms and corresponding ECG findings. (*A*) During normal sinus rhythm and in the absence of accessory or concealed pathways, electrical impulses (*gray arrows*) travel through the AV node using homogenous adjacent fibers. The result is narrow QRS complexes preceded by P waves, with regular P-R intervals. (*B*) When 2 adjacent pathways (alpha [α] and beta [β], *red arrows*) with different conduction and refractory periods lie within or near the AV node, a re-entry circuit might develop. The impulse uses one pathway for anterograde conduction and the other for retrograde conduction.

is masked. Because the circuit involves tissue above the bundle of His, the result is a narrow complex tachycardia.

Re-entry pathways can also be anatomically distinct. For example, when accessory conduction bundles exist, such as WPW syndrome, the impulse may use the normal conduction pathway for one limb of the loop (SA node → AV node → His bundle → right/left bundle branch → Purkinje fibers) and use the accessory bundle for the other limb of the loop (Purkinje fibers → atria → AV node), again, creating a circuit for the re-entry mechanism. Nevertheless, re-entry circuits can develop anywhere in the heart.[3,6,8] For example, when a circuit is completely residing in the atria, then atrial flutter/fibrillation may develop, but when it is completely residing in the ventricle, then ventricular tachycardia/fibrillation might develop.

The second most common type of PSVT is AV reciprocating tachycardia (AVRT). It includes WPW syndrome. AVRT occurs when there is a second conduction pathway that bypasses the AV node, thus dangerously and directly linking the atria and ventricles. WPW syndrome was first described in 1930 by cardiologists Louis Wolff, John Parkinson, and Paul Dudley White, thus, the name, Wolff-Parkinson-White syndrome. It is characterized by the presence of one or more accessory conduction pathways between the atria and the ventricles, referred to as the bundle of Kent.[11] During sinus rhythm, the bundle of Kent typically bypasses the normal physiologic delay of the AV node and results in the premature excitation of some parts of the ventricles before full depolarization through the right and left bundle branches and Purkinje fibers (**Fig. 2**A); this is manifested on the ECG by a slurred QRS onset (delta wave) resulting in a wide QRS complex.[8,12]

Usually, the accessory Kent pathway has a longer refractory period, and, hence, a critically timed premature atrial contraction can be blocked by the bundle of Kent, but

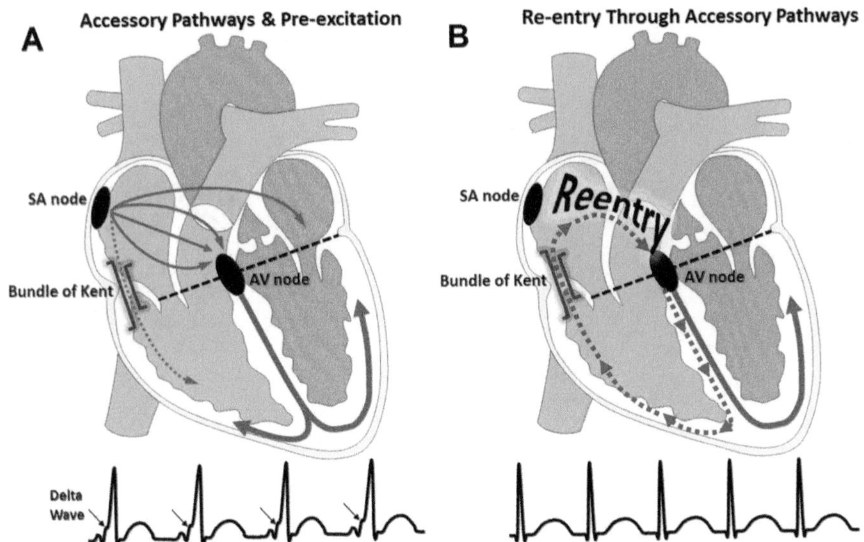

Fig. 2. Accessory pathways during sinus rhythm and during PSVT. (*A*) During normal sinus rhythm when an accessory pathway exists (eg, bundle of Kent, bars), the electrical impulse bypasses the AV node and results in premature excitation of the ventricles; the result is short P-R intervals with a delta wave that widens the QRS complex. (*B*) The accessory pathways typically have a longer refractory period, so a critically timed premature beat can be conducted through the AV node but not the accessory pathway. Upon the ventricular excitation, the accessory pathway is ready for excitation and is used for retrograde conduction and circuit formation (*dotted line*).

normally conducted through the right and left bundle branches and Purkinje fibers. By the time the ventricles are activated, the bundle of Kent is used for retrograde activation of the atrium, resulting in AVRT that appears on the ECG as a narrow QRS complex tachycardia (**Fig. 2**B).[9,12] In some instances, the bundle of Kent is capable of creating re-entry circuits through anterograde activation (the impulse passes anterograde through the accessory pathway to the ventricle first; then, in a retrograde direction through the bundle of His and the AV node). This phenomenon, even though uncommon, results in wide QRS complex PSVT that mimics ventricular tachycardia; thus, careful interpretation of the ECG is required.[13]

WPW-related accessory pathways are not common in the context of PSVT. However, nearly 30% of all PSVT cases are associated with other concealed accessory pathways.[5,6] These pathways are only capable of retrograde conduction and do not interfere with normal anterograde electrical conduction, which means that there are no electrocardiographic signatures associated with such pathways during sinus rhythm ("concealed"). When a concealed pathway contributes to a circuit formation as the retrograde limb of the circuit, PSVT can develop using a mechanism similar to that of AVRT.

CAUSE AND CLINICAL SIGNIFICANCE

PSVT is mainly attributed to the presence of abnormal conduction pathways, which can either include adjacent pathways (α and β channels seen in AVNRT) or structurally distinct pathways (AVRT seen with accessory or concealed bundles).[7,14,15] Although the exact cause for the presence of these pathways is not clear, women compared to men have a 2-fold increased risk of developing PSVT,[3] and WPW syndrome tends to have familial inheritance patterns.[7,12]

Another contributing mechanism is enhanced automaticity of the AV node. Factors that may enhance automaticity include (1) substance abuse (alcohol, nicotine, coffee, cocaine); (2) medications (digitalis toxicity, β-blockers, pseudoephedrine); and (3) psychological factors (stress, anxiety, panic attacks).[6] Although the inducibility of accessory pathways diminishes over time (AVRT is more common at younger ages), increased myocardial arrhythmogenicity places older adults (>65 years) at a 5-fold increased risk of developing AVNRT.[3]

ELECTROCARDIOGRAPHIC CHARACTERISTICS

A 12-lead ECG obtained during sinus rhythm and during an active episode of tachycardia is important in accurately diagnosing and identifying the cause of PSVT. AVNRT is characterized by a regular, narrow QRS complex tachycardia with no visible P waves (**Fig. 3**A), whereas AVRT is characterized by a regular, narrow complex tachycardia with a negative P wave (P-R interval <90 milliseconds; **Fig. 3**B) or a delayed P wave (R-P interval > P-R interval; **Fig. 3**C).[8,13]

During sinus rhythm, WPW is characterized by (1) a short PR interval of less than 120 milliseconds; (2) a slurring of an initial portion of the QRS complex (delta wave), which either interrupts the P wave or arises immediately after its termination; (3) a QRS duration greater than 120 milliseconds; and (4) secondary ST and T-wave changes (**Fig. 3**D). However, during episodes of PSVT, the ECG for those with pre-excitation would most likely resemble AVRT (see **Fig. 3**C).[16]

DIAGNOSTIC TESTING AND MANAGEMENT

In the absence of structural heart disease, most patients will have an unremarkable past medical history and physical examination. Therefore, initial evaluation should not only include a history and a physical examination, but also a resting 12-lead ECG.[5] A resting 12-lead ECG is important for defining the mechanism of the tachycardia and selection of proper treatment (treatments that target the AV node might not be effective in terminating non-AV node–dependent tachycardia).[3] Further diagnostic testing may be

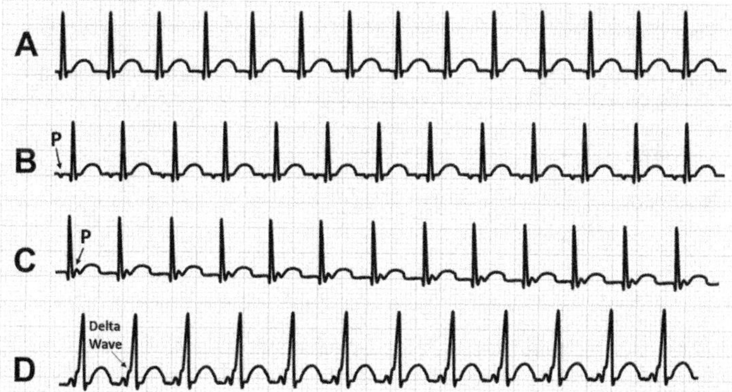

Fig. 3. Typical ECG findings according to type of PSVT. (*A*) ECG manifestations associated with AV nodal re-entry tachycardia. (*B, C*) AVRT and (*D*) WPW syndrome.

needed if initial evaluation suggests structural heart disease. Jugular venous distention, however, may suggest AVNRT due to atrial contraction against closed AV valves. Other differential diagnoses to consider while ruling out possible causes include electrolytes abnormalities, hyperthyroidism, and/or substance side effects (digoxin, pseudoephedrine, alcohol).

Emergency medical providers are typically the first to evaluate and treat patients with SVT regardless of cause. Current treatment guidelines are based on the recent 2015 recommendations by the American Heart Association and the American College of Cardiology (**Fig. 4**).[3] For hemodynamically stable patients with regular SVT (including PSVT), the first-line therapy is vagal maneuvers. Patients need to be taught these techniques because they are effective in terminating PSVT. However, the patient needs to perform these techniques early during an episode before a sympathetic response to PSVT is established. The Valsalva maneuver is the most effective technique, followed by carotid massage (for adults) and facial immersion in cold water (for children). However, in acute-care settings, intravenous adenosine is recommended for effective and rapid treatment of PSVT. Adenosine is an endogenous purine nucleoside that slows AV nodal conduction and results in transient AV nodal block; the recommended dose is 6 mg given intravenously, and therapeutic effects can be seen within 30 seconds of administration. If unsuccessful, intravenous diltiazem or verapamil can be used as an effective alternative therapy for the acute treatment of PSVT. Intravenous β-blockers should be used as a last option in these patients. Although some patients might present with wide-complex PSVT (WPW when the accessory pathway is used for anterograde conduction), test doses of adenosine, diltiazem, or verapamil are only recommended when PSVT is associated with narrow QRS complexes, which again emphasizes the importance of obtaining a 12-lead ECG before initiating any acute pharmacologic therapy.[5] If the above treatments are

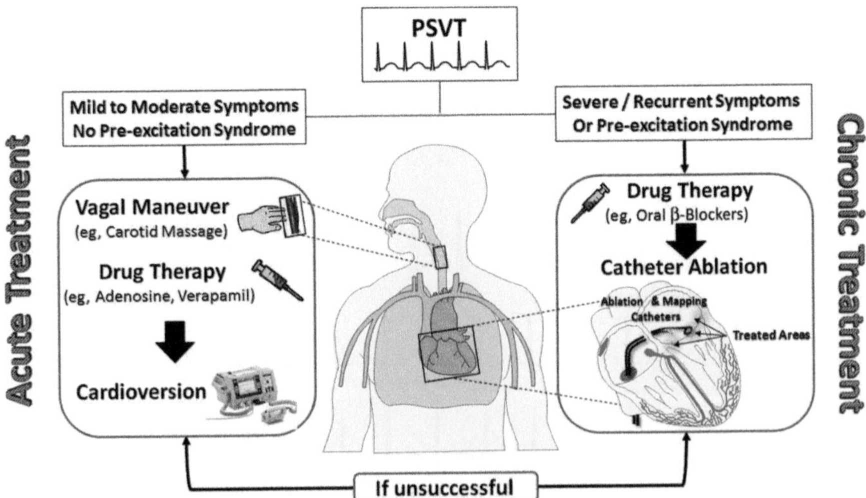

Fig. 4. Acute and chronic treatment of PSVT. Acute treatment includes the vagal maneuver and/or adenosine, followed by other class IV agents for the hemodynamically stable and/or synchronized cardioversion for the hemodynamically unstable. The chronic treatment of choice is catheter ablation or oral β-blockers, diltiazem, or verapamil for patients who are ineligible or who are reluctant to undergo invasive testing.

unsuccessful, or if the patient is hemodynamically unstable, synchronized cardioversion is recommended for the acute treatment of PSVT (see **Fig. 4**).

Many PSVT episodes are well tolerated and/or easily terminated and therefore do not require chronic therapy. However, for patients whose PSVT is not well tolerated (hemodynamic instability) or cannot be easily terminated, chronic drug treatment or catheter ablation is recommended.[3] Oral β-blockers, diltiazem, or verapamil can be useful in those with symptomatic PSVT without pre-excitation, whereas an electrophysiologic (EP) study with possible catheter ablation is recommended for those with pre-excitation during sinus rhythm (see **Fig. 4**). An EP study is an invasive procedure used to assess the heart's electrical activity and different conduction pathways. For example, the initial approach for ablation of AVNRT is targeted on the slow AV nodal pathway, whereas in the context of AVRT, the target for catheter ablation is the accessory pathway. If the patient is not a candidate for an ablation, or if the above agents are not effective, then either flecainide or propafenone is recommended for the ongoing management of PSVT followed by oral sotalol, dofetilide, amiodarone, or digoxin.[3]

PROGNOSIS

In the absence of pre-excitation or other structural heart disease, PSVT is generally non-life-threatening, and catheter ablation results in a permanent cure in most patients. However, despite the low incidence of life-threatening arrhythmias in WPW, current guidelines recommend risk stratification of these patients using EP testing to identify those deemed to be at high risk for future lethal arrhythmic events.[7] The latter group needs to be treated with catheter ablation, pacemakers, and/or implantable cardioverter-defibrillators. Nevertheless, some studies suggest that the presence of PSVT increases the future risk of stroke, independent of other demographic and clinical factors.[15]

Case study discussion

Dave's initial evaluation revealed no significant past medical or family history. His physical examination and ECG were normal (including no pre-excitation). The cardiologist diagnosed Dave with PSVT. Because the episode was aborted by splashing cold water on Dave's face, the cardiologist recommended, that should it occur again, trying a Valsalva maneuver. He also recommended that Dave track the frequency of the episodes, and if they became frequent or sustained, contacting the cardiologist for further evaluation and treatment strategies. For further risk stratification, a 24-hour Holter ECG recording could be ordered to track the frequency of PSVT episodes or to evaluate the presence of any other arrhythmias.

SUMMARY

PSVT is commonly diagnosed during adolescence and early adulthood. Symptoms may include palpitations, chest pain, shortness of breath, and/or dizziness. PSVT is rarely associated with structural heart disease and, hence, an initial physical examination and resting ECG are typically insignificant. Symptomatic patients are treated with vagal maneuvers and/or intravenous adenosine, and possibly with cardioversion if hemodynamically unstable. Patients with recurrent symptoms can be treated with long-term oral β-blockers, diltiazem, or verapamil. Radiofrequency catheter ablation is retained for those with severe recurrent symptoms or those with pre-excitation syndromes (WPW).

REFERENCES

1. Al-Zaiti S, Rittenberger JC, Reis SE, et al. Electrocardiographic responses during fire suppression and recovery among experienced firefighters. J Occup Environ Med 2015;57(9):938–42.
2. Al-Zaiti SS. Inflammation-induced atrial fibrillation: pathophysiological perspectives and clinical implications. Heart Lung 2015;44(1):59–62.
3. Page RL, Joglar JA, Caldwell MA, et al. 2015 ACC/AHA/HRS guideline for the management of adult patients with supraventricular tachycardia: executive summary: a report of the American College of Cardiology/American Heart Association Task Force on Clinical Practice Guidelines and the Heart Rhythm Society. Circulation 2016;133(14):e471–505.
4. Orejarena LA, Vidaillet H, DeStefano F, et al. Paroxysmal supraventricular tachycardia in the general population. J Am Coll Cardiol 1998;31(1):150–7.
5. Ferguson JD, DiMarco JP. Contemporary management of paroxysmal supraventricular tachycardia. Circulation 2003;107(8):1096–9.
6. Lowenstein SR, Halperin BD, Reiter MJ. Paroxysmal supraventricular tachycardias. J Emerg Med 1996;14(1):39–51.
7. Al-Khatib SM, Arshad A, Balk EM, et al. Risk stratification for arrhythmic events in patients with asymptomatic pre-excitation: a systematic review for the 2015 ACC/AHA/HRS guideline for the management of adult patients with supraventricular tachycardia: a report of the American College of Cardiology/American Heart Association Task Force on clinical practice guidelines and the Heart Rhythm Society. Circulation 2016;133(14):e575–86.
8. Macfarlane P, Lawrie V. Comprehensive electrocardiology, theory and practice in health and disease. New York: Pergamon Press; 1989.
9. Durrer D, Schoo L, Schuilenburg R, et al. The role of premature beats in the initiation and the termination of supraventricular tachycardia in the Wolff-Parkinson-White syndrome. Circulation 1967;36:644–62.
10. Wu D, Denes P, Amat-Y-Leon F, et al. Clinical, electrocardiographic and electrophysiologic observations in patients with paroxysmal supraventricular tachycardia. Am J Cardiol 1978;41(6):1045–51.
11. Wolff L, Parkinson J, White PD. Bundle-branch block with short P-R interval in healthy young people prone to paroxysmal tachycardia. Am Heart J 1930;5(6):685–704.
12. Munger TM, Packer DL, Hammill SC, et al. A population study of the natural history of Wolff-Parkinson-White syndrome in Olmsted County, Minnesota, 1953-1989. Circulation 1993;87(3):866–73.
13. Surawicz B, Knilans T, editors. Chou's electrocardiography in clinical practice. 6th edition. Philadelphia: WB Saunders Company; 2008.
14. Obeyesekere MN, Leong-Sit P, Massel D, et al. Risk of arrhythmia and sudden death in patients with asymptomatic preexcitation: a meta-analysis. Circulation 2012;125(19):2308–15.
15. Kamel H, Elkind MS, Bhave PD, et al. Paroxysmal supraventricular tachycardia and the risk of ischemic stroke. Stroke 2013;44(6):1550–4.
16. Surawicz B, Childers R, Deal BJ, et al. AHA/ACCF/HRS recommendations for the standardization and interpretation of the electrocardiogram: part III: intraventricular conduction disturbances: a scientific statement from the American Heart Association Electrocardiography and Arrhythmias Committee, Council on Clinical Cardiology; the American College of Cardiology Foundation; and the Heart Rhythm Society endorsed by the International Society for Computerized Electrocardiology. J Am Coll Cardiol 2009;53(11):976–81.

Ventricular Tachycardias

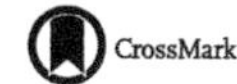

Characteristics and Management

Aksana Baldzizhar, MD[a,*], Ekaterina Manuylova, MD[b,c], Roman Marchenko, MD[d], Yury Kryvalap, MD[e], Mary G. Carey, PhD, RN[a,f]

KEYWORDS

• Ventricular tachycardias • Torsades de pointes • Electrocardiogram • Arrhythmia • Nursing

KEY POINTS

- When possible, a resting 12-lead electrocardiogram (ECG) should be recorded during ventricular arrhythmia to optimize the correct diagnosis.
- One of the challenges of ventricular arrhythmias is accurate and rapid interpretation of an ECG.
- It is important to distinguish torsades de pointes from other forms of ventricular tachycardias because the management of it is different.

INTRODUCTION

Nearly half a million people die annually in the United States from sudden cardiac death (SCD), often due to ventricular tachycardias (VTs). The most common types of arrhythmias leading to primary cardiac arrest and SCD are VT, ventricular fibrillation (VFIB), and torsades de pointes (TdP) (**Table 1**).[1–4] VT is characterized by abnormal electrical impulses that originate in the ventricular conduction system, ischemic myocardium, or scar tissue. As a result, these electrical impulses spread through the myocardium of ventricles and can either cross the atrioventricular (AV) node, capturing the atria retrograde, or bypass it (ventriculoatrial dissociation). Arrhythmogenic factors include changes in autonomic nervous system activity, metabolic disturbances, and myocardial

Disclosure Statement: None of the authors has any conflicts to disclose.

[a] School of Nursing, University of Rochester Medical Center, 601 Elmwood Avenue, Box 619-7, Rochester, NY 14642, USA; [b] Department of Endocrinology, Diabetes and Metabolism, University of Rochester, 601 Elmwood Avenue, Box 693, Rochester, NY 14642, USA; [c] Department of Medicine, Strong Memorial Hospital, University of Rochester Medical Center, 601 Elmwood Avenue, Box-693, Rochester, NY 14642, USA; [d] Department of Interventional Electrophysiology, Federal Center of Cardiovascular Surgery, 6, Stasova Street, Penza 440071, Russia; [e] Department of Pathology, Strong Memorial Hospital, University of Rochester Medical Center, 601 Elmwood Avenue, Box-626, Rochester, NY 14642, USA; [f] Department of Nursing Practice, Strong Memorial Hospital, University of Rochester Medical Center, 601 Elmwood Avenue, Box 619-7, Rochester, NY 14642, USA

* Corresponding author.

E-mail address: aksana_baldzizhar@urmc.rochester.edu

Crit Care Nurs Clin N Am 28 (2016) 317–329
http://dx.doi.org/10.1016/j.cnc.2016.04.004 ccnursing.theclinics.com
0899-5885/16/$ – see front matter © 2016 Elsevier Inc. All rights reserved.

Table 1
Cardiac arrest arrhythmias and survival in hospitalized patients

	Pulseless VT (%)	VFIB (%)	PEA (%)	Asystole (%)
Total cardiac arrests in adults by first documented cardiac arrest rhythm	7.4	10.0	54.6	28.0
Survival to discharge of adults by first documented cardiac arrest rhythm	44.9	46.2	19.8	20.2

Abbreviation: PEA, pulseless electrical activity.

Data from Neumar RW, Eigel B, Callaway CW, et al. American Heart Association response to the 2015 Institute of Medicine report on strategies to improve cardiac arrest survival. Circulation 2015;132(11):1049–70.

ischemia due to coronary artery disease as well as proarrhythmic actions of cardiac and noncardiac drugs.[2,5–7] Many patients exhibiting VT have underlying structural heart disease that leads to abnormal electrical automaticity.[8–10]

VTs can be induced by an excitation wave re-entry mechanism. It occurs either in a localized area (micro-re-entry) or in a wider area of myocardium (macro-re-entry). Other mechanisms of re-entry include abnormal automaticity, triggered activity, or a combination of the above factors. A resting 12-lead electrocardiogram (ECG) should be recorded during the ventricular arrhythmia to optimize the correct diagnosis.[2,11] One of the challenges is accurate and rapid interpretation of an ECG[3,11,12] because clinical management of ventricular arrhythmias is often complicated by the need for extremely rapid diagnosis and treatment.[4,13–15] Thus, the purpose of this article is to review the criteria of the diagnoses and management of VTs. In addition, the pathophysiology and ECG characteristics of nonsustained VT (NSVT), VT, VFIB, and TdP are discussed (**Fig. 1**).

NONSUSTAINED VENTRICULAR TACHYCARDIA

NSVT is characterized by a rapid heart rate of at least 120 bpm with at least 3 or more consecutive ventricular beats in fewer than 30 seconds.[2] Among the ventricular

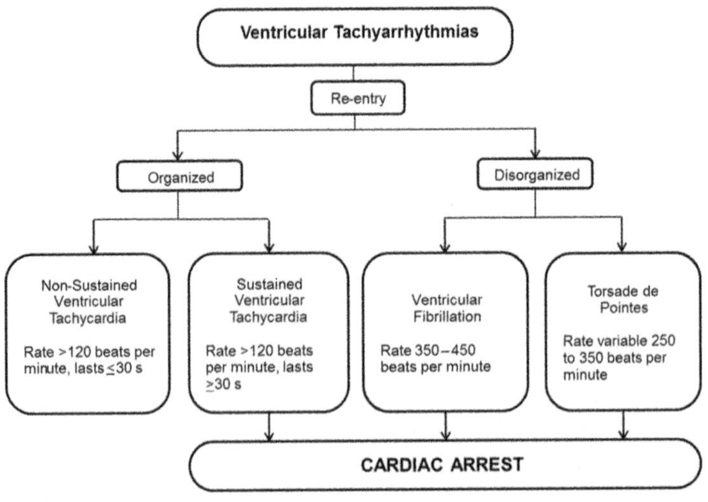

Fig. 1. The 4 types of VTs.

arrhythmias, NSVT does not substantially compromise the cardiac output because it is short-lasting. Often the patient is asymptomatic, but NSVT can be detected during hospital bedside cardiac monitoring or ambulatory Holter monitoring. Symptom severity depends on heart rate and duration of the NSVT. Any heart rate greater than 150 bpm compromises the AV synchrony of the heart, by dramatically reducing filling time of the ventricles, and therefore, resulting in a compromised cardiac output. Although premature ventricular contractions may precede NSVT suggesting myocardial irritability, NSVT may suddenly appear and disappear. Patients may experience palpitations, dizziness, chest pain, and fainting. Importantly, NSVT may serve as a potential marker for development of VT and SCD. NSVT in patients with structural heart disease has a more serious prognosis than in patients with absence of cardiac abnormalities[16,17] because this type of VTs indicates predisposition to development of more severe and even fatal arrhythmias.[18]

Predisposing causes leading to NSVT include the following[16,19–22]:

- Structural heart disease: coronary heart disease, hypertrophic cardiomyopathy, and, rarely, nonischemic cardiomyopathy, mitral valve prolapse, mitral regurgitation, and aortic stenosis.
- Electrolyte abnormalities.
- VT syndromes.

ECG characteristics of NSVT include the following:

- Three or more consecutive ventricular beats.
- A rate of greater than 120 bpm.
- A duration of less than 30 seconds (**Fig. 2**).[6]

Management

The presence of NSVT serves as a significant marker of possible heart disease. If underlying heart disease is subsequently discovered, treatment should be directed toward this abnormality. If no underlying heart disease is found, monitoring may be optional. The management includes oxygen via nasal cannula, electrolyte replacement (potassium and magnesium) if needed, and, in rare cases, antiarrhythmic medications.[16] In patients with structurally normal hearts, β-blockers and calcium channel blockers can be used because class IC agents (flecainide and propafenone) are not effective. Patients with coronary artery disease benefit from class III antiarrhythmic agents such as amiodarone and sotalol. Another consideration is catheter ablation for patients with highly symptomatic and drug refractory of idiopathic NSVT, especially exercise-induced NSVT.[23,24]

Sequence of Actions

Sequence of actions for SVT is not an emergency, so therapy may not be indicated if ejection fraction (EF) is normal. Patients with a reduced EF of 35% may be candidates for an implantable cardioverter-defibrillator (ICD) because better survival has been reported among ICD patients than with patients using conventional antiarrhythmic drugs.[13]

SUSTAINED VENTRICULAR TACHYCARDIA

Sustained VT has almost the same characteristics as NSVT but lasts more than 30 seconds.[2] An ectopic focus sends its impulses to the ventricles causing repeated ventricular contractions in a regular rapid fashion; these impulses depolarize the ventricles bypassing the normal conduction pathways (**Fig. 3**).

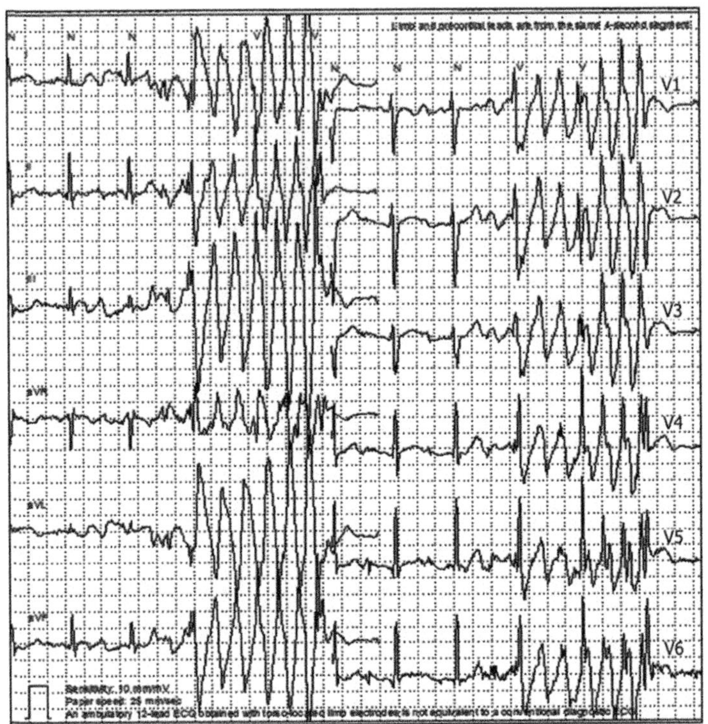

Fig. 2. NSVT. A 12-lead ECG of sinus tachycardia. The heart rate is 130 bpm and is NSVT.

Predisposing causes leading to VT include the following[19,25]:

- VT usually occurs in patients with significant structural heart disease: coronary artery disease with a history of myocardial infarction, dilated cardiomyopathy, hypertrophic cardiomyopathy, mitral valve prolapse, aortic stenosis, complex congenital heart disease, cardiac sarcoidosis, and arrhythmogenic right ventricular cardiomyopathy/dysplasia. In this setting, VT possesses a high risk for SCD.
- Less often, VT can occur in grossly normal-appearing hearts; however, in these cases the heart abnormalities are still present but subtle. This group of VT syndromes includes repetitive monomorphic VT, paroxysmal sustained VT, and idiopathic left VT.

Underlying pathophysiology includes inherited abnormalities of cardiac ion channels or structural proteins. Clinical manifestations of VT depend on the ventricular rate, the presence of underlying heart disease, and the degree of left ventricular systolic dysfunction. Symptoms vary widely from discomfort in the heart area to SCD. Faster heart rates, greater than 180 bpm, may cause drops in arterial pressure and be a cause of syncope due to decreased cardiac output. Hemodynamic instability is defined as hypotension that results in poor peripheral perfusion and leads to dizziness, angina, presyncope/syncope, cardiogenic shock, or seizures. Sustained VT can progress to VFIB and SCD.[17,21]

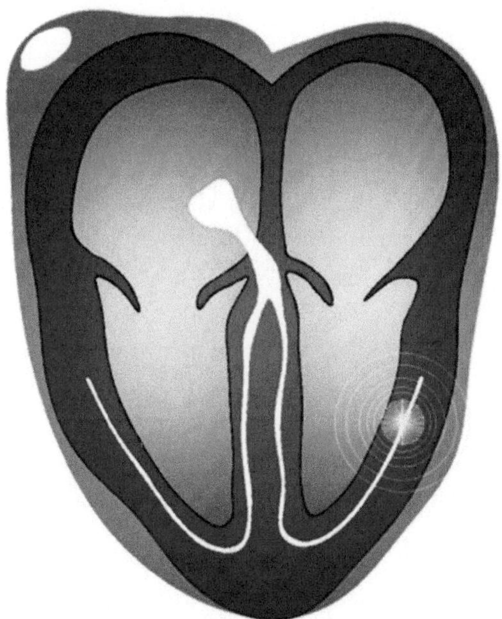

Fig. 3. VT foci originate in the ventricle, and retrograde depolarization occurs.

Electrocardiogram Characteristics

- VT is a regular rhythm with wide and abnormal QRS complexes of at least 0.12 seconds in duration with the heart rate greater than 120 bpm for at least 30 seconds[6,26] (**Fig. 4**).
- A 12-lead ECG verifies the diagnosis of VT, and the presence of Q waves or fragmentation of the QRS complex suggests underlying structural heart disease.[27,28]

Management

- Monomorphic VT and polymorphic VT, specifically TdP, are both life threatening. Identification of a VT subtype on an ECG is important in choosing the correct treatment strategy.[13–15,18,23,29]
- A hemodynamically stable patient with a palpable pulse and regular rhythm requires oxygen, electrolyte replacement, and administration of antiarrhythmic agents such as amiodarone, lidocaine, and procainamide.
- A hemodynamically unstable patient (mean arterial pulse <60 mm Hg), with a palpable pulse, requires synchronized cardioversion followed by the administration of procainamide, amiodarone, or sotalol. In pulseless VT cases, cardiopulmonary resuscitation (CPR) includes immediate defibrillation followed by the administration of vasopressin or epinephrine. If the pulse does not restore, amiodarone, lidocaine, or magnesium is indicated. Of survivors of VT who suffered from hemodynamic instability, structural heart disease, or have an EF, less than 30% are candidates for an ICD placement. The use of an ICD prevents sudden death and improves survival in patients.[19,30]

Sequence of Actions

1. Assess the patient for arrhythmia (the heart rate is typically at least 150 bpm in tachyarrhythmia).[19,29,31,32]

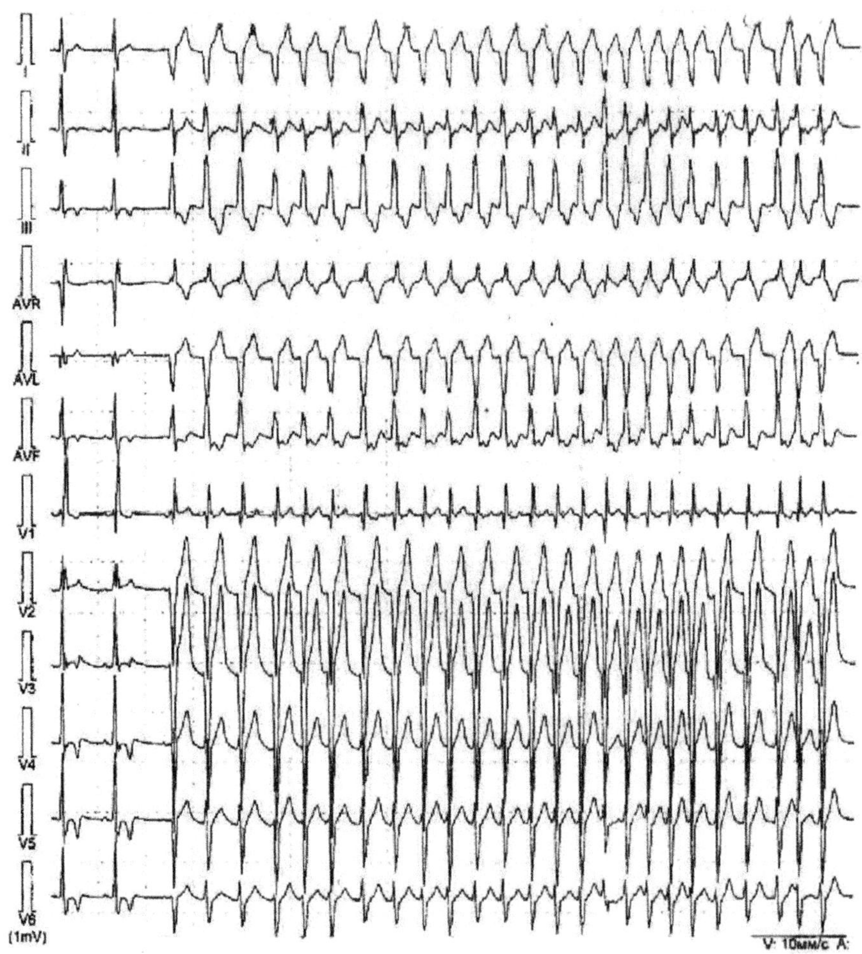

Fig. 4. Sustained VT. A 12-lead ECG of sustained VT; heart rate is 107 bpm.

2. Palpate pulse, pulse present.
3. Activate emergency medical services (EMS) and assess patient.
4. Maintain patient's airway; assist breathing as necessary.
5. Monitor arterial oxygen saturation and give oxygen if hypoxic.
6. Insert an intravenous (IV) catheter.
7. Monitor rhythm, blood pressure, and pulse oximetry.
8. Identify and correct any electrolyte abnormalities.
9. Assess for persistent tachycardia consequences and complications: hypotension, acutely altered mental status, signs of shock, ischemic chest discomfort, acute heart failure, and so on.
10. If there are no VT complications and the patient is stable, IV infusion of an antiarrhythmic agent is recommended: amiodarone 150 mg over 10 minutes and repeated doses as needed if VT recurs, follow-up with maintenance infusion of 1 mg/min for the first 6 hours. Procainamide or sotalol can also be used (procainamide 20–50 mg/min) until arrhythmia terminates, hypotension ensues, the QRS

duration prolongs by at least 50%, or a maximum dose of 17 mg/kg is reached. Maintenance infusion is 1 to 4 mg/min. Procainamide is contraindicated in chronic heart failure. The sotalol IV dose is 100 mg (1.5 mg/kg) over 5 minutes. Avoid the use of procainamide and sotalol in prolonged QT interval presence. Patients with unstable tachyarrhythmia are treated with synchronized cardioversion (the protocol is described in later discussion).

VENTRICULAR FIBRILLATION

VFIB is uncoordinated chaotic contractions of individual fibers and muscle groups initiated by disorganized depolarization (**Fig. 5**). Ventricular myocardium becomes nonresponsive to stimuli generated in the sinus node. The heart is essentially quivering with completely ineffective contractions so cardiac output is absent, and the patient suffers from hemodynamic collapse with subsequent cardiac arrest.

Predisposing causes leading to VFIB include the following[23,25,33]:

- Ischemic heart disease: coronary artery disease with myocardial infarction or angina, coronary artery embolism, nonatherogenic coronary artery disease (arteritis, dissection, congenital coronary artery anomalies), coronary artery spasm;
- Nonischemic heart disease: congenital heart disease, hypertrophic cardiomyopathy, dilated cardiomyopathy, valvular heart disease, arrhythmogenic right ventricular dysplasia, myocarditis, acute pericardial tamponade, acute myocardial rupture, aortic dissection;
- Nonstructural heart disease: idiopathic VFIB, Brugada syndrome, long QT syndrome, Wolff-Parkinson-White syndrome, complete heart block, familial SCD, chest-wall trauma with myocardial contusion;
- Noncardiac disease: pulmonary embolism, obstruction of central airways, intracranial hemorrhage, drowning, Pickwickian syndrome, drug-induced, sudden infant death syndrome.

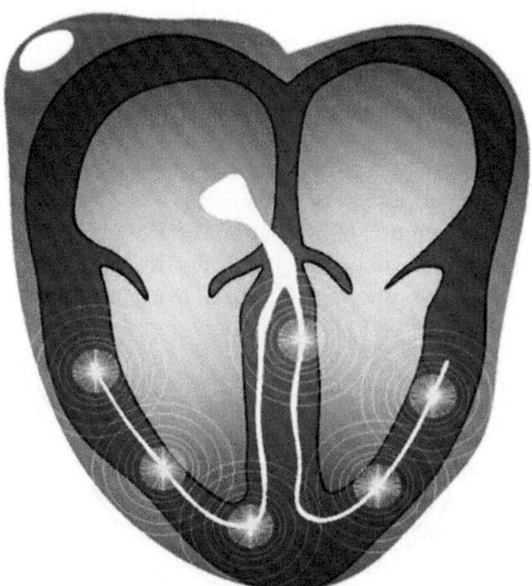

Fig. 5. VFIB multifoci originate in the ventricle, and retrograde depolarization occurs.

VFIB causes the collapse and loss of consciousness followed by the absence of pulse and/or heartbeat[23] and results from multiple localized areas of micro-re-entry without any organized electrical activity; importantly, VFIB is a lethal rhythm and; if not addressed promptly, leads to cardiac death.[18]

Electrocardiogram Characteristics

- VFIB is a rapid disorganized ventricular rhythm with a rate of 350 to 450 bpm and a shapeless QRS complex and T wave. There is a complete absence of properly formed QRS complexes and no obvious P waves.[6,26]

Management

- An unwitnessed VFIB case: CRP followed by immediate defibrillation using a nonsynchronized mode
- A witnessed VFIB case: immediate defibrillation using a nonsynchronized mode, CPR, administration of vasopressin, epinephrine, amiodarone, lidocaine, and magnesium[16,29,34]

Sequence of Actions

1. Assess the patient.[19,32,34–36]
2. Palpate pulse; pulse not present.
3. Activate EMS and assess patient.
4. Start CPR, deliver oxygen, and attach monitor/defibrillator.
5. Assess whether heart rhythm is shockable, and shock if applicable. If so, shock energy is biphasic or monophasic. Biphasic energy is manufacturer recommended to be delivered in an initial dose of 120 to 200 J; second and subsequent doses should be equivalent, and higher doses may be considered. Monophasic energy is delivered at 360 J. Repetitive, lower-energy biphasic waveform shock has an equal or higher success for eradicating VFIB than defibrillators that increase the current with each shock (200 J, 300 J, and 360 J).
6. Continue CPR for 2 minutes; begin drug treatment. Drug treatment includes epinephrine IV/intraosseous infusion dose (1 mg every 3–5 minutes), vasopressin IV dose (40 units can replace first or second dose of epinephrine), amiodarone IV dose (first dose is 300 mg bolus, and second dose is 150 mg).
7. If no effect, assess whether heart rhythm is shockable, and use shock if advised.
8. Continue CPR for 2 minutes and drug treatment. Consider advanced airway. Advanced airway includes endotracheal intubation (ET) and use waveform capnography to monitor ET tube placement, deliver 8 to 10 breaths per minute with continuous effective chest compressions.
9. If not effective, assess whether heart rhythm is shockable, and shock if applicable.
10. Continue CPR for 2 minutes; use amiodarone and treat reversible causes, including: hypovolemia, hypoxia, hypothermia, acidosis, hypokalemia/hyperkalemia, tamponade, tension pneumothorax, toxins, coronary or pulmonary thrombosis.
11. Continue and repeat steps 7 to 10.

Knowledge of and skills in advanced cardiac live support are necessary in a hospital, because first responders and nurses have to be prepared to quickly apply defibrillator pads and defibrillate a patient without waiting for a doctor if the situation requires it. Importantly, decreased survival is directly linked to a delay greater than 10 seconds.[37] Once defibrillator pads are placed, chest compression should be continued uninterrupted except for rhythm assessment and the actual defibrillation. Although protection of the airways is important, the chest compressions should have the higher priority. In adults, target chest compressions to ventilation ratio should be 30 compressions to 2 ventilations, without the presence of an advanced airway. Excessive ventilation may lead to decreased survival. Excessive ventilation leads to increased intrathoracic chest pressure, decreased venous return, and decreased coronary perfusion pressure.[37–41]

Torsades de Pointes

In French, "torsades de pointes" means "twisting of the spikes." This arrhythmia is an atypical form of VT that is difficult to classify.[3,6] Dessertenne[42] presented the first scientific description of TdP in 1966 with his theory of its mechanism.[26] In TdP, the ECG is characterized by the absence of discernible QRS complexes and T waves. The dysrhythmia is associated with a long QT syndrome and accompanied by no cardiac output. TdP often manifests with syncope, especially in women,[43] and is potentially lethal. Importantly, TdP is strongly associated with medication and electrolyte imbalances that delay repolarization, so a clinical priority is to identify precipitating factors that may contribute to the arrhythmia.

Predisposing causes leading to TdP include the following[44,45]:

- Prolonged QT syndrome: associated with congenital anomaly, bradycardia, or complete heart block;
- Quinidine or procainamide toxicity;
- Tricyclic overdose;
- Malnutrition;
- Electrolyte disturbances, especially hypokalemia, hypomagnesemia, and hypocalcemia;
- Heart diseases, especially cardiomyopathies, myocardial infarction, and myocarditis.

Electrocardiogram Characteristics

- QRS complexes are bizarre, sharply pointed spikes that shift or twist around the isoelectric line. The rate is a variable and very rapid at 250 to 350 bpm[6,26] (**Fig. 6**).

Management

- Discontinuation of any precipitating agents and aggressive correction of metabolic abnormalities, such as hypokalemia or hypomagnesemia, is an initial step. IV magnesium sulfate is a main therapy, being highly effective for the

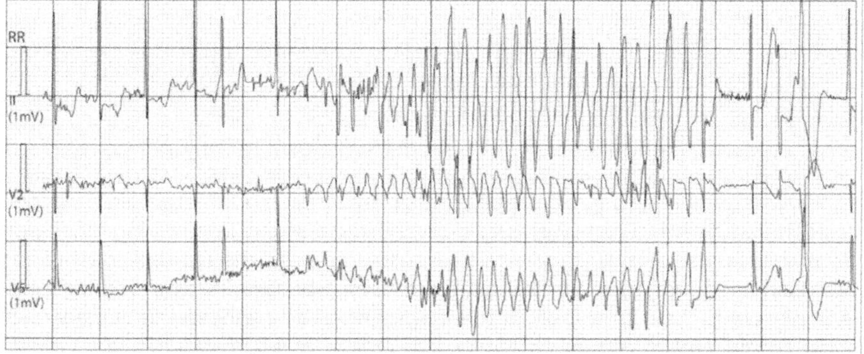

Fig. 6. An ECG of intermittent TdP. Leads II, V2, and V5 show shockable atrial flutter worsening into TdP and recovering with sinus rhythm and a premature ventricular contractions.

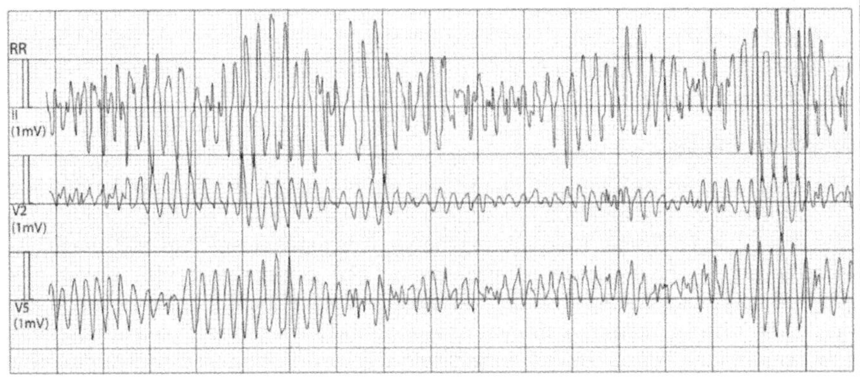

Fig. 7. An ECG of sustained TdP. Leads II, V2, V5.

treatment of this rhythm disturbance. If a patient deteriorates, immediate defibrillation should be attempted.[16,34,46]

Sequence of Actions

1. Assess the patient.[19,32,34,46]
2. Palpate pulse, pulse weak or not present.
3. Activate EMS.
4. Start CPR, deliver oxygen, and attach monitor/defibrillator.
5. Discontinue any precipitating agents.
6. Correct metabolic abnormalities, such as hypokalemia and hypomagnesemia by giving 1 to 2 g of magnesium sulfate administered IV over 1 to 2 minutes followed by a maintenance infusion of 1 to 2 g per hour.
7. Continue to monitor cardiac rhythm, blood pressure, and pulse oximetry.
8. If noneffective (**Fig. 7**) and the patient deteriorates, immediately use cardiac defibrillation.
9. If the TdP converts to VFIB, the treatment modalities include the continuation of defibrillation and antiarrhythmic agents as described in earlier discussion.

SUMMARY

VTs can be suddenly lethal without high-quality care; therefore, timely diagnoses and management are crucial because they improve survival rates. The key points are that the initiation of high-quality CPR, early defibrillation, and the avoidance of excessive ventilation are essential. A physical examination and a resting 12-lead ECG are used to diagnose ventricular arrhythmias. Given its asymptomatic nature, NSVT is typically diagnosed during cardiac monitoring or an exercise stress test. Most patients with VT have underlying cardiac disease, which is associated with a worse prognosis when compared with patients without structural heart disease. Importantly, many ventricular arrhythmias quickly lead to cardiac arrest. Assessment and treatment of VTs depend on 2 factors: patient status (stable vs unstable) and the type of arrhythmia. It is important to distinguish TdP from other forms of VT because the management of it is different. Health care providers should carefully monitor for ventricular arrhythmias and be ready to respond quickly and effectively to reduce complications and prevent SCD.

REFERENCES

1. Cleverley K, Mousavi N, Stronger L, et al. The impact of telemetry on survival of in-hospital cardiac arrests in non-critical care patients. Resuscitation 2013;84(7): 878–82.
2. Goldberger JJ, Cain ME, Hohnloser SH, et al. American Heart Association/ American College of Cardiology Foundation/Heart Rhythm Society scientific statement on noninvasive risk stratification techniques for identifying patients at risk for sudden cardiac death: a scientific statement from the American Heart Association Council on Clinical Cardiology Committee on electrocardiography and arrhythmias and council on epidemiology and prevention. Circulation 2008;118(14):1497–518.
3. Carey MG, Al-Zaiti SS, Canty JM Jr, et al. High-risk electrocardiographic parameters are ubiquitous in patients with ischemic cardiomyopathy. Ann Noninvasive Electrocardiol 2012;17(3):241–51.
4. Neumar RW, Eigel B, Callaway CW, et al. American Heart Association response to the 2015 Institute of Medicine report on strategies to improve cardiac arrest survival. Circulation 2015;132(11):1049–70.
5. Liu BR, Cherry EM. Image-based structural modeling of the cardiac Purkinje network. Biomed Res Int 2015;2015:621034.
6. Wagner GS, Strauss DG. Marriott's practical electrocardiography. Philadelphia: Wolters Kluwer Health; 2013.
7. Priori SG, Aliot E, Blomstrom-Lundqvist C, et al. Task force on sudden cardiac death of the European Society of Cardiology. Eur Heart J 2001;22(16):1374–450.
8. Bloom HL. Treatment of ventricular tachycardia: consider ablation sooner. F1000 Med Rep 2009;1:71–5.
9. Sacher F, Tedrow UB, Field ME, et al. Ventricular tachycardia ablation: evolution of patients and procedures over 8 years. Circ Arrhythm Electrophysiol 2008;1(3): 153–61.
10. Richardson K, Engel G, Yamazaki T, et al. Electrocardiographic damage scores and cardiovascular mortality. Am Heart J 2005;149(3):458–63.
11. Shen MJ, Zipes DP. Role of the autonomic nervous system in modulating cardiac arrhythmias. Circ Res 2014;114(6):1004–21.
12. Tan SY, Sungar GW, Myers J, et al. A simplified clinical electrocardiogram score for the prediction of cardiovascular mortality. Clin Cardiol 2009;32(2):82–6.
13. Moss AJ, Hall WJ, Cannom DS, et al. Improved survival with an implanted defibrillator in patients with coronary disease at high risk for ventricular arrhythmia. Multicenter automatic defibrillator implantation trial investigators. N Engl J Med 1996; 335(26):1933–40.
14. Raitt MH, Renfroe EG, Epstein AE, et al. "Stable" ventricular tachycardia is not a benign rhythm: insights from the Antiarrhythmics Versus Implantable Defibrillators (AVID) registry. Circulation 2001;103(2):244–52.
15. Singh JP, Hall WJ, McNitt S, et al. Factors influencing appropriate firing of the implanted defibrillator for ventricular tachycardia/fibrillation: findings from the multicenter automatic defibrillator implantation trial II (MADIT-II). J Am Coll Cardiol 2005;46(9):1712–20.
16. European Heart Rhythm Association, Heart Rhythm Society, Zipes DP, et al. ACC/AHA/ESC 2006 guidelines for management of patients with ventricular arrhythmias and the prevention of sudden cardiac death: a report of the American College of Cardiology/American Heart Association Task Force and the European Society of Cardiology Committee for practice guidelines

(Writing Committee to Develop Guidelines for Management of Patients with Ventricular Arrhythmias and the Prevention of Sudden Cardiac Death). J Am Coll Cardiol 2006;48(5):e247–346.

17. Perez MV, Dewey FE, Tan SY, et al. Added value of a resting ECG neural network that predicts cardiovascular mortality. Ann Noninvasive Electrocardiol 2009; 14(1):26–34.
18. Al-Zaiti SS, Carey MG. The prevalence of clinical and electrocardiographic risk factors of cardiovascular death among on-duty professional firefighters. J Cardiovasc Nurs 2015;30(5):440–6.
19. Zipes DP, Camm AJ, Borggrefe M, et al. ACC/AHA/ESC 2006 guidelines for management of patients with ventricular arrhythmias and the prevention of sudden cardiac death: a report of the American College of Cardiology/American Heart Association task force and the European Society of Cardiology Committee for practice guidelines (writing committee to develop guidelines for management of patients with ventricular arrhythmias and the prevention of sudden cardiac death): developed in collaboration with the European Heart Rhythm Association and the Heart Rhythm Society. Circulation 2006;114(10):e385–484.
20. Wolfe RR, Driscoll DJ, Gersony WM, et al. Arrhythmias in patients with valvar aortic stenosis, valvar pulmonary stenosis, and ventricular septal defect. Results of 24-hour ECG monitoring. Circulation 1993;87(2 Suppl):I89–101.
21. Monserrat L, Elliott PM, Gimeno JR, et al. Non-sustained ventricular tachycardia in hypertrophic cardiomyopathy: an independent marker of sudden death risk in young patients. J Am Coll Cardiol 2003;42(5):873–9.
22. Marine JE, Shetty V, Chow GV, et al. Prevalence and prognostic significance of exercise-induced nonsustained ventricular tachycardia in asymptomatic volunteers: BLSA (Baltimore Longitudinal Study of Aging). J Am Coll Cardiol 2013; 62(7):595–600.
23. American College of Physicians. MKSAP 15: medical knowledge self-assessment program. Philadelphia: American College of Physicians; 2009.
24. Pedersen CT, Kay GN, Kalman J, et al. EHRA/HRS/APHRS expert consensus on ventricular arrhythmias. Europace 2014;16(9):1257–83.
25. Belhassen B, Viskin S. Idiopathic ventricular tachycardia and fibrillation. J Cardiovasc Electrophysiol 1993;4(3):356–68.
26. Dubin DB. Rapid interpretation of EKG's: an interactive course. Tampa (FL): Cover Publ.; 2000.
27. Das MK, Khan B, Jacob S, et al. Significance of a fragmented QRS complex versus a Q wave in patients with coronary artery disease. Circulation 2006; 113(21):2495–501.
28. Das MK, Suradi H, Maskoun W, et al. Fragmented wide QRS on a 12-lead ECG: a sign of myocardial scar and poor prognosis. Circ Arrhythm Electrophysiol 2008; 1(4):258–68.
29. Callaway CW, Soar J, Aibiki M, et al. Part 4: advanced life support: 2015 International Consensus on Cardiopulmonary Resuscitation and Emergency Cardiovascular Care Science with Treatment Recommendations. Circulation 2015;132(16 Suppl 1):S84–145.
30. Epstein AE, Dimarco JP, Ellenbogen KA, et al. ACC/AHA/HRS 2008 guidelines for device-based therapy of cardiac rhythm abnormalities. Heart Rhythm 2008;5(6): e1–62.
31. Nolan JP, Hazinski MF, Aickin R, et al. Part 1: executive summary: 2015 International Consensus on Cardiopulmonary Resuscitation and Emergency

Cardiovascular Care Science with Treatment Recommendations. Resuscitation 2015;95:e1–31.

32. Neumar RW, Otto CW, Link MS, et al. Part 8: adult advanced cardiovascular life support: 2010 American Heart Association guidelines for cardiopulmonary resuscitation and emergency cardiovascular care. Circulation 2010;122(18 Suppl 3): S729–67.
33. Alings M, Wilde A. "Brugada" syndrome: clinical data and suggested pathophysiological mechanism. Circulation 1999;99(5):666–73.
34. Sinz E, Navarro K, American Heart Association. Advanced cardiovascular life support: provider manual. Dallas (TX): American Heart Association; 2011.
35. National Clinical Guideline Centre. Atrial fibrillation: the management of atrial fibrillation. London (United Kingdom): PubMed Health, US National Library of Medicine; 2014.
36. Yousuf O, Chrispin J, Tomaselli GF, et al. Clinical management and prevention of sudden cardiac death. Circ Res 2015;116(12):2020–40.
37. Kupchik N, Bridges E. Improving outcomes from in-hospital cardiac arrest. Am J Nurs 2015;115(5):51–4.
38. Herlitz J, Svensson L. Prehospital care soon to be routine in suspected acute coronary syndrome. Lakartidningen 2001;98(35):3696–8 [in Swedish].
39. Sell RE, Sarno R, Lawrence B, et al. Minimizing pre- and post-defibrillation pauses increases the likelihood of return of spontaneous circulation (ROSC). Resuscitation 2010;81(7):822–5.
40. Herlitz J, Bang A, Aune S, et al. Characteristics and outcome among patients suffering in-hospital cardiac arrest in monitored and non-monitored areas. Resuscitation 2001;48(2):125–35.
41. Wiegand DJLMH. AACN procedure manual for critical care. St. Louis (MO): Elsevier Health Sciences; 2013.
42. Dessertenne F. Ventricular tachycardia with two variable opposing foci. Arch Mal Coeur Vaiss 1966;59:263–72.
43. Task Force for the Diagnosis and Management of Syncope, European Society of Cardiology (ESC), European Heart Rhythm Association (EHRA), et al. Guidelines for the diagnosis and management of syncope (version 2009). Eur Heart J 2009; 30(21):2631–71.
44. Maisel WH, Kuntz KM, Reimold SC, et al. Risk of initiating antiarrhythmic drug therapy for atrial fibrillation in patients admitted to a university hospital. Ann Intern Med 1997;127(4):281–4.
45. Straus SM, Sturkenboom MC, Bleumink GS, et al. Non-cardiac QTc-prolonging drugs and the risk of sudden cardiac death. Eur Heart J 2005;26(19):2007–12.
46. Tzivoni D, Banai S, Schuger C, et al. Treatment of torsade de pointes with magnesium sulfate. Circulation 1988;77(2):392–7.

Cardiac Monitoring in the Emergency Department

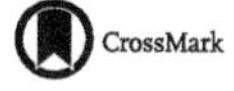

Jessica K. Zègre-Hemsey, PhD, RN[a,*], J. Lee Garvey, MD[b], Mary G. Carey, PhD, RN[c]

KEYWORDS

- Emergency department • Cardiac monitoring • Arrhythmias
- Myocardial ischemia/ infarction • 12-Lead electrocardiogram
- ST-Segment monitoring • QT-Interval

KEY POINTS

- Emergency department (ED) care demands rapid, accurate diagnosis and stabilization of patients with time-sensitive conditions such as acute myocardial infarction and arrhythmia.
- Cardiac monitoring strategies in the ED include standard 12-lead electrocardiography and bedside monitoring for arrhythmias and myocardial ischemia.
- Electrocardiographic signs of myocardial ischemia drive clinical decision making such as the activation of cardiac catheterization of patients with ST-elevation myocardial infarction.

INTRODUCTION

More than 8 million patients with chest pain and/or anginal equivalent symptoms present to emergency departments (ED) each year, accounting for the second, most common cause of ED visits for adults.[1] Cardiovascular emergencies account for approximately 10% of all ED visits.[1,2] ED clinicians are required to rapidly differentiate between life-threatening conditions and non–life-threatening ones and accurately determine which course of treatment will result in optimal patient outcomes.[3] Cardiac monitoring strategies, which include 12-lead electrocardiography (ECG) and bedside monitors, enable clinicians to detect arrhythmias, myocardial ischemia, and QT-interval measurements in real time.

Cardiac monitoring was first introduced nearly 60 years ago for critically ill patients, but today is used increasingly to monitor ED patients with a variety of conditions. Early monitoring focused on heart rate measurement and fatal arrhythmia detection.[4] Today, monitoring has expanded to include diagnoses of complex arrhythmias, acute myocardial ischemia, and pharmacologically induced prolonged QT intervals.[5]

Disclosures: Nothing to disclose (J.K. Zègre-Hemsey, M.G. Carey); Philips Healthcare (J.L. Garvey).
[a] School of Nursing, University of North Carolina at Chapel Hill, Carrington Hall, Campus Box 7460, Chapel Hill, NC 27599-7460, USA; [b] Carolinas Medical Center, 1000 Blythe Boulevard, Charlotte, NC 28203, USA; [c] Clinical Nursing Research Center, School of Nursing, Strong Memorial Hospital, University of Rochester Medical Center, 601 Elmwood Avenue, Box 619-7, Rochester, NY 14642, USA
* Corresponding author.
E-mail address: jzhemsey@email.unc.edu

Crit Care Nurs Clin N Am 28 (2016) 331–345
http://dx.doi.org/10.1016/j.cnc.2016.04.009 ccnursing.theclinics.com
0899-5885/16/$ – see front matter © 2016 Elsevier Inc. All rights reserved.

Emergency nurses are often the first care providers to evaluate patients presenting to the ED; therefore, they are pivotal in determining the urgency of initiating cardiac monitoring for risk stratification of patients arriving in the ED. Emergency nurses require ongoing education and training on equipment because cardiac monitoring technologies are evolving rapidly to meet the demands of complex, patient care. This paper describes current cardiac monitoring practices in an ED setting, with a primary focus on arrhythmia, myocardial ischemia, and QT-interval monitoring.

Cardiac monitoring is a useful, noninvasive diagnostic tool to monitor the wide array of patient conditions in the ED. To assist clinicians in determining which patients need monitoring, experts in electrocardiology and cardiac monitoring convened to develop practice standards for hospital ECG monitoring.[4,6] These practice standards encompass all areas of hospital cardiac monitoring, including arrhythmia, myocardial ischemia, and QT interval monitoring. Guidelines reflect expert opinions based on clinical experience and research; however, data for best practices for hospital cardiac monitoring are limited.[6] Conditions common to the ED setting and implications for cardiac monitoring are discussed; each is categorized by the rating system below, which was developed by the American College of Cardiology Emergency Cardiac Care Committee for cardiac monitoring.[4]

Class I: Cardiac monitoring is indicated in most, if not all, patients in this group.
Class II: Cardiac monitoring may be beneficial to some patients but not considered essential for all patients.
Class III: Cardiac monitoring is not indicated because a patient's risk of a serious event is so low that monitoring has no therapeutic monitoring benefit.

ARRHYTHMIA MONITORING IN THE EMERGENCY DEPARTMENT

Arrhythmias frequently reflect underlying diseases and comorbidities, and are detected by clinicians as well as computer algorithms in cardiac monitors, which are set to trigger an alarm when a life-threatening arrhythmia is detected.[7] **Box 1** lists conditions for which arrhythmia monitoring may be beneficial (class II) or unnecessary (class III).[4,6] However, ED patients at significant risk for immediate fatal arrhythmias, such as ventricular fibrillation (**Fig. 1**) or asystole, should receive continuous cardiac monitoring (class I).

Cardiac Arrest

Patients resuscitated from cardiac arrest should be monitored continuously for arrhythmias in the ED because they are at high risk for recurring arrhythmias. A cardiac monitor/defibrillator should be attached to the patient on arrival in the ED to ascertain underlying rhythm and monitoring should continue until the cause of the event is known, and/or until an implantable defibrillator is in place.[4] Patients recovering from cardiac arrest should also have continuing cardiac monitoring if required to leave the ED for diagnostic or therapeutic procedures or are transported to the intensive care unit for admission.[6]

Acute Coronary Syndrome

Accelerated diagnostic protocols have been developed to discern low-risk from high-risk patients presenting to the ED with chest pain.[1] Risk stratification for patients with suspected acute coronary syndrome (ACS) includes prompt arrhythmia and ischemia monitoring on ED arrival, serial 12-lead ECG acquisition, and cardiac biomarker testing over a 6- to 12-hour period.[1,4] Patients with negative results are deemed low risk and receive a confirmatory study, for example, exercise and treadmill testing,

Box 1
Recommendations for cardiac arrhythmia monitoring in the emergency department

Class I conditions

1. Patients resuscitated from cardiac arrest.
2. Patients in the early phase of acute coronary syndrome.
3. Patients with newly diagnosed high-risk coronary lesions.
4. Patients after cardiac surgery.
5. Patients after implantation of automatic defibrillator or pacemaker lead who are pacemaker dependent.
6. Patients with temporary or transcutaneous pacemaker.
7. Patients with AV block (Wenckebach, Mobitz II, complete block, new-onset bundle branch block in the setting of myocardial infarction).
8. Patients with arrhythmia complicating Wolff–Parkinson–White syndrome with rapid conduction over an accessory pathway.
9. Patients with drug-induced long-QT syndrome.
10. Patients with acute heart failure, pulmonary edema.
11. Patients with major trauma, acute respiratory failure, sepsis, shock, pulmonary embolus, major noncardiac surgery, drug overdose, or other indications for intensive care.
12. Patients who require conscious sedation or anesthesia for diagnostic/therapeutic procedures.
13. Patients with any hemodynamically unstable arrhythmia.
14. Patients with syncope owing to underlying heart condition.
15. Pediatric patients diagnosed with any arrhythmia.

Class II conditions

1. Patients with subacute heart failure.
2. Patients with do not resuscitate orders.

Class III conditions

1. Patients with chronic, rate-controlled atrial fibrillation.
2. Obstetric patients, unless heart disease is present.

Adapted from Drew BJ, Califf RM, Funk M, et al. Practice standards for electrocardiographic monitoring in hospital settings: an American Heart Association scientific statement from the Councils on Cardiovascular Nursing, Clinical Cardiology, and Cardiovascular Disease in the Young: endorsed by the International Society of Computerized Electrocardiology and the American Association of Critical-Care Nurses. Circulation 2004;110(17):2721–46; and Drew BJ, Funk M. Practice standards for ECG monitoring in hospital settings: executive summary and guide for implementation. Crit Care Nurs Clin North Am 2006;18(2):157–68.

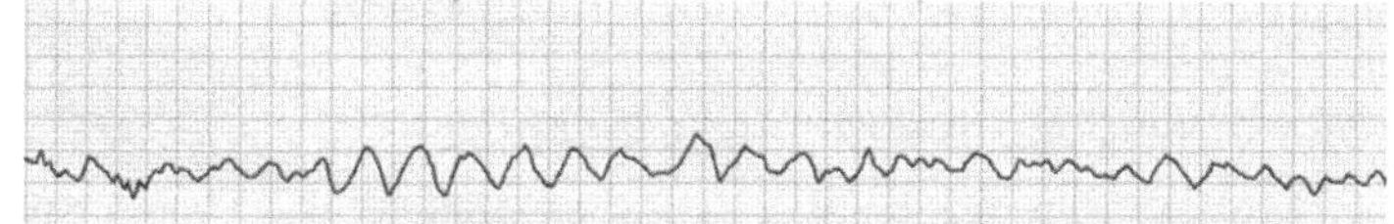

Fig. 1. Example of ventricular fibrillation, a class I condition in arrhythmia monitoring.

before discharge.[1] Alternatively, high-risk patients with acute myocardial infarction who undergo early reperfusion therapy in the prehospital period or in the ED are at risk for malignant reperfusion arrhythmias. These patients should receive uninterrupted, arrhythmia monitoring during both interhospital and intrahospital transport.[4] Arrhythmia monitoring is also indicated for patients with newly diagnosed, critical left main coronary artery disease and other high-risk coronary lesions who are candidates for urgent revascularization. Patients with unstable angina should undergo cardiac monitoring until infarction is ruled out and signs that transient ECG changes and symptoms are absent.[4]

Recently, Winkler and colleagues[8] studied 278 patients diagnosed with ACS to determine the potential benefits of ST-segment monitoring in the ED; they found the incidence of ventricular arrhythmias (premature ventricular contractions, nonsustained ventricular tachycardia, and malignant arrhythmias) over the first 24 hours of hospitalization to be lower than studies conducted before the reperfusion era in the late 1980s.

Heart Failure and/or Pulmonary Edema

Continuous arrhythmia monitoring is recommended for patients with signs and symptoms of heart failure and/or pulmonary edema. Acute heart failure is a major risk factor for atrial and ventricular arrhythmias, and some therapies such as intravenous positive inotropic drugs have significant proarrhythmic properties.[4]

Atrioventricular Block

Patients who present to the ED with palpitations, syncope, dizziness, or lightheadedness may be experiencing an atrioventricular (AV) block; ongoing arrhythmia monitoring is indicated for patients with Mobitz I or Mobitz II (second-degree AV block), complete heart block (third-degree AV block), or new-onset, bundle branch block in the setting of acute myocardial infarction.[4] ECG monitoring should continue until the block resolves or definitive therapy (a permanent pacemaker) is implemented.

After Cardiac Surgery

Patients presenting to the ED after cardiac surgery should be monitored for arrhythmias because they are at risk for developing ventricular tachycardia or fibrillation, AV block, and sinus node dysfunction.[4] Moreover, the incidence of postoperative atrial fibrillation is 32% after coronary artery bypass surgery, 64% after combined bypass and mitral valve replacement surgery, 49% after combined bypass and aortic valve replacement, and 11% after heart transplantation.[9,10] Emergency nurses should consider that the onset of atrial fibrillation typically occurs on the second to fourth postoperative days, and that a majority of these patients are asymptomatic.[4,11]

Syncope

Patients presenting to the ED with syncope of truly unknown origin should receive arrhythmia monitoring because heart disease is a major predictor of death and/or fatal arrhythmia in syncopal patients.[4] Patients should be monitored until an arrhythmic cause has been ruled out by electrophysiologic testing or other evaluation is completed.

ISCHEMIA MONITORING IN THE EMERGENCY DEPARTMENT

Coronary heart disease is the leading cause of death in the United States and becoming the most frequent cause of death worldwide.[12,13] Coronary heart disease is characterized by stable and unstable periods, the latter reflects progression of occlusion in a coronary artery and manifests as ACS. ACS is a spectrum of time-sensitive clinical syndromes that includes (1) unstable angina, (2) non–ST-segment elevation myocardial infarction, and (3) ST-segment elevation myocardial infarction.[14] Prompt diagnosis and effective early management of ACS in the ED are imperative because numerous clinical trials have established that a more aggressive approach to the treatment of myocardial ischemia improves patient outcomes.[4,14,15] If left undetected, ACS results in devastating outcomes such as myocardial infarction, heart failure, and death.[15–17] Strategies to prevent infarction or reduce infarct size rely heavily on the ability of clinicians to identify myocardial ischemia in the ED. Cardiac monitoring enables clinicians to identify rapidly patients who require urgent intervention from those with benign conditions who can be discharged home.[1,14,18,19]

The 12-Lead Electrocardiogram

To date, the 12-lead ECG remains the gold standard used for initial screening, identifying, and evaluating patients with chest pain and anginal equivalents.[20] The ECG is the most widely used initial diagnostic test because it is ubiquitous, noninvasive, and inexpensive, and provides vital information about cardiac rhythm, presence of arrhythmias, myocardial ischemia/infarction, and other abnormalities.[15,21,22] The American College of Cardiology, The American Heart Association, and The European Society of Cardiology recommend that all patients who present to the ED with chest pain have a 12-lead ECG recorded within 10 minutes of arrival.[23–26] This recommendation is based on the premise that longer delays are associated with worse outcomes, and ST-segment pattern recognition shortens the delay between the first medical contact and life-saving reperfusion therapies.[15,23,27]

The standard 12-lead ECG uses 10 electrodes to record the electrical activity of the heart. Six precordial leads are placed across the precordium in anatomically specific locations and 3 limb leads may be placed either (1) on the distal limbs, the preferred placement, for standard, resting 12-lead ECG acquisition, or (2) where the limbs attach to the torso (Mason-Likar) for continuous ECG monitoring, such as exercise testing (**Fig. 2**).[28] Using different limb lead placements produces a similar, but not identical, 12-lead ECG; different limb lead placement between serial ECGs may result in waveform morphology changes that computer algorithms falsely interpret as myocardial ischemia.[4,6] Therefore, emergency nurses should receive ongoing training and education about the importance of correct and standardized electrode placement for accurate cardiac monitoring.[29]

Electrocardiographic Signs of Ischemia

Changes in the intracellular action potential in myocardial ischemia, injury, and infarction result in changes in ECG waveforms. ECG changes indicating ischemia (**Fig. 3**) include ST-elevation, ST-depression, or T-wave inversion and occur before myocardial infarction, providing the ability to intervene to restore blood flow before myocardial cell death ensues. The presence of acute ischemic changes on the initial ECG, often conducted at presentation to the ED, is associated with a higher risk of cardiac events.[30] Acute ischemic changes are unpredictable and dynamic in nature, which suggests that a single snap-shot 12-lead ECG is inadequate, and continuous or serial ECG monitoring is superior diagnostically.[20,31–33] The presence of ischemic signs may advise the ED clinicians to activate the catheterization laboratory for patients suffering from acute myocardial infarction; this extends into the prehospital period where paramedics may analyze ECGs acquired in the ambulance and activate the catheterization laboratory before hospital arrival.[34]

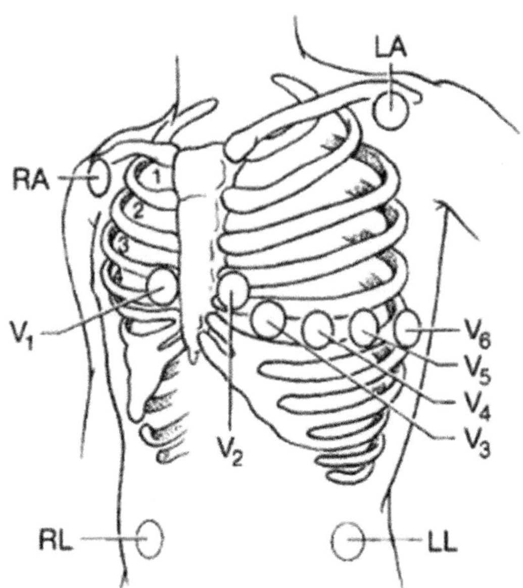

Fig. 2. Mason-Likar electrode placement for continuous 12-lead electrocardiographic monitoring. LA, left arm; LL, left leg; RA, right arm; RL, right leg. (*From* Zegre Hemsey J. Optimizing pre-hospital electrocardiography to improve the early diagnosis of acute coronary syndrome. San Francisco (CA): University of California; 2011; with permission.)

Universal ECG criteria for myocardial infarction were developed to increase the sensitivity and specificity of the ECG by recognizing gender, age, and lead differences.[35] Electrocardiographic criteria (in the absence of left ventricular hypertrophy and left bundle branch block) include:

- ST elevation at the J-point in 2 contiguous leads with the cutpoints: 0.2 mV or greater in men 40 years or older; 0.25 mV or greater in men less than 40 years, or 0.15 mV or greater in women in leads V_2 to V_3 and/or 0.1 mV or greater in all other leads.
- ST-depression and T-wave changes defined by new horizontal or down-sloping ST depression 0.05 mV or greater in 2 contiguous leads and/or T inversion 0.1 mV or greater in 2 contiguous leads with prominent R wave or R/S ratio of greater than 1.

Emergency nurses or technicians typically obtain the initial ECG in the ED, which is interpreted by an emergency physician or cardiologist. Because of the decreasing mentoring of physicians to learn ECG interpretation, there has been a recent call for the training of cardiovascular nurse practitioners to interpret ECG.[36] This is an important consideration in the ED setting, where clinicians rely on interdisciplinary teamwork to manage the large array of patients with cardiac complaints.

Serial Electrocardiographic Monitoring

Serial ECG acquisition is recommended when the initial ECG is nondiagnostic, but patient signs or symptoms are consistent with acute myocardial infarction.[27]

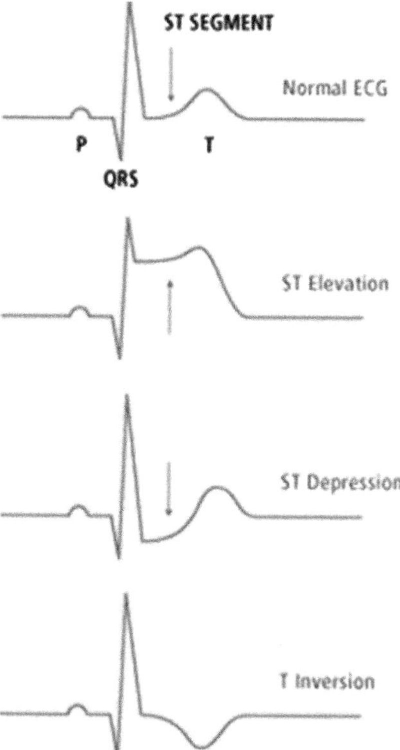

Fig. 3. Changes in the electrocardiograph (ECG) in the ST-segment indicative of myocardial ischemia and infarction. (*From* Zegre Hemsey J. Optimizing pre-hospital electrocardiography to improve the early diagnosis of acute coronary syndrome. San Francisco (CA): University of California; 2011; with permission.)

Current guidelines specifically recommend the initial ECGs be repeated at 5- to 10-minute intervals if the initial ECG is not diagnostic but the patient remains symptomatic and a high clinical suspicion for ACS persists.[37] Prior studies suggest that serial ECG recordings enhance the diagnostic sensitivity for ACS as compared with abnormalities on a single tracing and offer the opportunity for clinicians to observe changes between tracings that may be more difficult to interpret individually, enabling detection of evolving changes of ischemia that, by nature, are dynamic and unpredictable.[31] Serial ECG comparisons should be made using the same recording technique because differences in waveform morphology have been observed between differing electrode configurations (eg, standard vs Mason-Likar placement).[6]

Continuous ST-Segment Monitoring in the Emergency Department

The American College of Cardiology/The American Heart Association guidelines recommend continuous bedside ST-segment monitoring for patients with a nondiagnostic initial ECG as an alternative to serial 12-lead ECGs.[38] Patients with ACS are the highest priority for ST-segment monitoring until they remain event free for 12 to 24 hours. Practice standards for ECG monitoring recommend continuous

ST-segment monitoring in (class I) patients for 8 to 12 hours in combination with serum biomarker testing to determine treatment priority in ED patients with suspected ACS or at risk for ACS.[4,18,39] Conversely, patients with left ventricular hypertrophy, left bundle branch block, ventricular pacing, and those with intermittent right bundle branch block may not necessarily benefit from ST-segment monitoring (class III) because these conditions present secondary ST/T-wave abnormalities that confound interpretation and may trigger false ST-segment alarms.[40]

ST-segment analysis software became available on bedside monitors in the mid 1980s, and is widely available in the United States.[39] However, surveys suggest that ST-segment monitoring software is not activated routinely by nurses because of lack of education, generations of numerous false alarms, and difficulty of use.[4,41] Moreover, the standard 12-lead ECG is not always convenient for continuous monitoring,[4] especially in the ED where patients are on gurneys, moved frequently to accommodate patient flow, and transported for diagnostic testing. Improvements to the user interface may help this situation.

Studies examining the value of ST-segment monitoring in the ED are limited. Fesmire and colleagues[32] examined the usefulness of ST-segment monitoring with serial ECG acquisition in 1000 patients with chest pain in the ED. Serial ECGs with ST-segment monitoring had greater sensitivity (68% vs 55%; $P<.0001$) and specificity (99 vs 97; $P<.01$) for detecting ACS compared with the initial "snapshot" ECG acquired on ED arrival. More recently, Bovino and colleagues[18] examined the value of bedside continuous ST-segment monitoring 163 patients with risk-stratified chest pain in the ED at intermediate risk for ACS. Investigators found no difference in detection of ischemia/infarction, time to diagnosis, or 30-day adverse events among patients before and after ST-segment monitoring implementation.[18] Further research is required to establish evidence-based guidelines for ST-segment monitoring in the ED setting.

Reduced Lead Sets

Reduced lead set technology enables synthesis of a 12-lead ECG from a small number of leads/electrodes, which makes continuous cardiac monitoring more feasible in the ED.[4] The EASI 5-lead system (Philips IntelliVue, Andover, MA) was the first derived 12-lead ECG and was developed by Dower[42] in 1988; it mathematically derives an ECG from 4 recording electrodes and a reference electrode (**Fig. 4**). Importantly, the derived 12-lead ECG is comparable with the standard 12-lead ECG for diagnosis of acute myocardial ischemia and wide complex QRS tachycardias, each of which requires multiple leads for accurate interpretation.[4,43,44]

Fig. 5 shows another commonly used 5-lead configuration for cardiac monitoring in the ED. Four limb electrodes and a fifth chest electrode can be placed in any of the standard precordial (V_1–V_6) positions; the chest electrode allows for recording of a true V lead, which may enhance the accuracy for arrhythmia detection.[4] However, this derived lead configuration is not sensitive for detection of myocardial ischemia.

QT INTERVAL MONITORING

Acute lengthening of the QT interval, an indirect measure of ventricular repolarization, can be observed in multiple clinical situations and is associated with syncope and sudden death from torsade de pointes (TdP).[4] TdP is a malignant polymorphic ventricular tachycardia that resembles ventricular fibrillation; it may self-terminate or progress to cardiac arrest and sudden cardiac death (**Fig. 6**).[4,7,45]

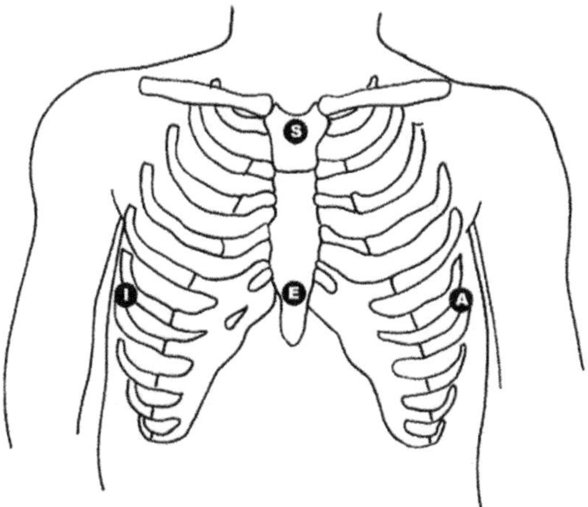

Fig. 4. EASI lead system electrode placement. The fifth ground electrode (not shown) may be placed anywhere on the body. (*From* Sejersten M, Pahlm O, Pettersson J, et al. Comparison of EASI-derived 12-lead electrocardiograms versus paramedic-acquired 12-lead electrocardiograms using Mason-Likar limb lead configuration in patients with chest pain. J Electrocardiology 2006;39(1):13–21.)

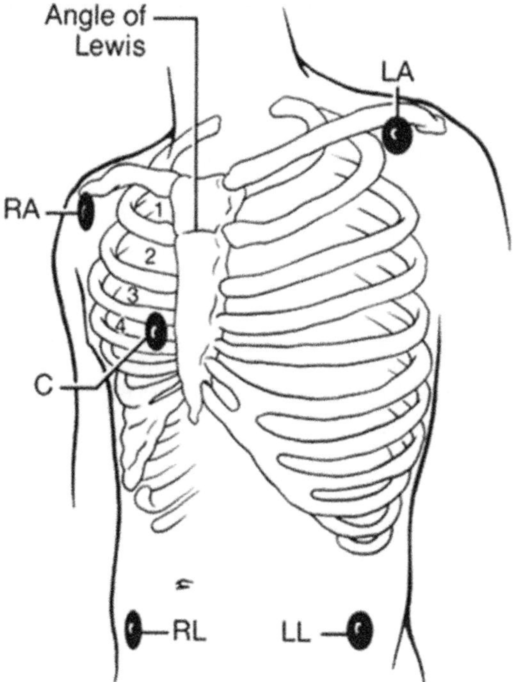

Fig. 5. Standard 5-electrode lead system in the emergency department. LA, left arm; LL, left leg; RA, right arm; RL, right leg. (*From* Drew BJ, Califf RM, Funk M, et al. Practice standards for electrocardiographic monitoring in hospital settings: an American Heart Association scientific statement from the Councils on Cardiovascular Nursing, Clinical Cardiology, and Cardiovascular Disease in the Young: endorsed by the International Society of Computerized Electrocardiology and the American Association of Critical-Care Nurses. Circulation 2004;110(17):2721–46.)

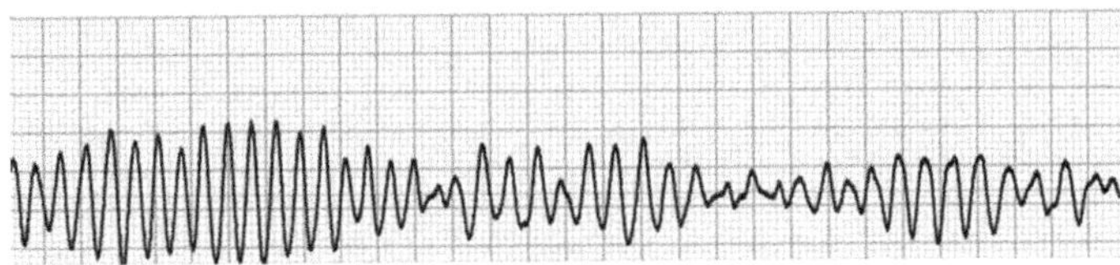

Fig. 6. Torsade de pointes is a lethal arrhythmia.

Typical features of TdP include (1) changes in amplitude and morphology of QRS complexes around the isoelectric line and (2) drug-induced TdP episodes that begin with a short-long-short pattern of R-R cycles consisting of a short premature ventricular complex followed by a compensatory pause and another premature ventricular complex.[46] A normal corrected QT (QT_c) for women is less than 0.46 seconds and for men is less than 0.45 seconds; a QT_c of greater than 0.50 seconds in either gender positively correlates with a higher risk for TdP. The duration of a QT_c is a reliable indicator of risk of cardiac events; therefore, patients with long QT syndrome and associated ventricular arrhythmias should receive QT monitoring in the ED (class I recommendation).[4,45]

The importance of QT monitoring in the ED cannot be underestimated because ED patients are uniquely at risk for developing TdP owing to their vast array of chief complaints and high acuity.[45] Specific patient characteristics are associated with development of TdP (**Box 2**) and should be considered during triage and risk stratification.[45]

Practice guidelines recommend measuring patients' QT/QT_c interval at baseline and documenting repeat measures at least once every 8 hours.[4,45] Patients in the ED may initially require QT/QT_c monitoring more frequently, especially if receiving medications (**Box 3**) known to prolong the QT interval.[45] Therefore, it is important for emergency nurses to acquire the knowledge, skill, and judgment to tailor QT/QT_c monitoring to individual patient needs.[45] Specific indications for QT interval monitoring of ED

Box 2
Characteristics of patients at risk for developing torsade de pointes

1. Women
2. Elderly
3. Heart disease
4. Acute neurologic events
5. Bradyarrhythmias with long pauses
6. Electrolyte disturbances (hypomagnesia, hypokalemia)
7. Malnutrition
8. Polypharmacy
9. Genetics (long QT syndrome, family history of sudden cardiac death, syncope)
10. Renal/hepatic dysfunction

Adapted from Pickham D, Drew BJ. QT/QTc interval monitoring in the emergency department. J Emerg Nurs 2008;34(5):428–34; with permission.

Box 3
Medications raising patient-risk of torsade de pointes

Generic Name	Clinical Use
Amiodarone	Antiarrhythmic
Amiodarone	Anticancer
Azithromycin	Antibiotic
Chlorpromazine	Antipsychotic/antiemetic
Ciprofloxacin	Antibiotic
Cocaine	Local anesthetic
Disopyramide	Antiarrhythmic
Dofetilide	Antiarrhythmic
Dronedarone	Antiarrhythmic
Droperidol	Antipsychotic/antiemetic
Erythromycin	Antibiotic
Flecainide	Antiarrhythmic
Haloperidol	Antipsychotic
Ibutilide	Antiarrhythmic
Levofloxacin	Antibiotic
Methadone	Opioid agonist
Ondansetron	Antiemetic
Quinidine	Antiarrhythmic
Sotalol	Antiarrhythmic
Thioridazine	Antipsychotic

Data from Arizona CERT. Available at: www.qtdrugs.org. Accessed December 14, 2015.

patients are listed in **Box 4**. Practice guidelines recommend that QT monitoring should continue until (1) the culprit drug is discontinued and/or decreased and no further prolonged QT_c is noted, (2) no further QT-related arrhythmias occur, (3) definitive therapy (permanent pacemaker) is established, and/or (4) electrolyte disorder has been corrected.[4,6,40]

Emergency nurses are in a unique position to identify and measure the QT interval on 12-lead ECGs acquired in the ED; they can be empowered with the knowledge of applying correction formulas to determine the QT_c, which accounts for the influence of heart rate.[45] Moreover, ED nurses can learn to interpret and document QT measurements when provided by the standard 12-lead ECG machine to optimize management of patients at possible risk for TdP.

Box 4
Indications for QT interval monitoring

1. Patients started on antiarrhythmic drug known to cause torsade de pointe (disopyramide, dofetilide, ibutilide, procainamide quinidine, sotalol).
2. Patients who overdose from proarrhythmic agents.
3. Patients with new onset bradyarrhythmias (complete heart block, long sinus pauses).
4. Patients with severe hypokalemia or hypomagnesemia.

Adapted from Pickham D, Drew BJ. QT/QTc interval monitoring in the emergency department. J Emerg Nurs 2008;34(5):429; with permission.

SUMMARY

The ED is a fast-paced, dynamic, and chaotic setting that requires quick and accurate decision making to distinguish high-acuity patients. The priority for emergency clinicians is to recognize and stabilize patients with emergent cardiovascular conditions that include, but are not limited to, myocardial ischemia/infarction and potentially life-threatening arrhythmias. Cardiac monitoring is one of the most commonly used diagnostic practices in the ED, and emergency nurses are poised to use valuable information revealed in ECG waveforms for early triage and risk stratification. Future research is needed to drive evidenced-based monitoring practices specific to patients in the ED.

REFERENCES

1. Amsterdam EA, Kirk JD, Bluemke DA, et al. Testing of low-risk patients presenting to the emergency department with chest pain: a scientific statement from the American Heart Association. Circulation 2010;122(17):1756–76.
2. Centers for Disease Control and Prevention. National Hospital Ambulatory Medical Care Survey: 2011 emergency department summary, vol. 386. Atlanta (GA): Centers for Disease Control and Prevention; 2011.
3. O'Connor RE, Al Ali AS, Brady WJ, et al. Part 9: acute coronary syndromes: 2015 American Heart Association guidelines update for cardiopulmonary resuscitation and emergency cardiovascular care. Circulation 2015;132(18 Suppl 2): S483–500.
4. Drew BJ, Califf RM, Funk M, et al. Practice standards for electrocardiographic monitoring in hospital settings: an American Heart Association scientific statement from the Councils on Cardiovascular Nursing, Clinical Cardiology, and Cardiovascular Disease in the Young: endorsed by the International Society of Computerized Electrocardiology and the American Association of Critical-Care Nurses. Circulation 2004;110(17):2721–46.
5. Drew BJ, Harris P, Zegre-Hemsey JK, et al. Insights into the problem of alarm fatigue with physiologic monitor devices: a comprehensive observational study of consecutive intensive care unit patients. PLoS One 2014;9(10):e110274.
6. Drew BJ, Funk M. Practice standards for ECG monitoring in hospital settings: executive summary and guide for implementation. Crit Care Nurs Clin North Am 2006;18(2):157–68.
7. Priori SG, Blomstrom-Lundqvist C, Mazzanti A, et al. 2015 ESC guidelines for the management of patients with ventricular arrhythmias and the prevention of sudden cardiac death: the task force for the management of patients with ventricular arrhythmias and the prevention of sudden cardiac death of the European Society of Cardiology (ESC) endorsed by: association for European Paediatric and Congenital Cardiology (AEPC). Eur Heart J 2015;36(41):2793–867.
8. Winkler C, Funk M, Schindler DM, et al. Arrhythmias in patients with acute coronary syndrome in the first 24 hours of hospitalization. Heart Lung 2013;42(6): 422–7.
9. Creswell LL, Schuessler RB, Rosenbloom M, et al. Hazards of postoperative atrial arrhythmias. Ann Thorac Surg 1993;56(3):539–49.
10. Thoren E, Hellgren L, Stahle E. High incidence of atrial fibrillation after coronary surgery. Interact Cardiovasc Thorac Surg 2016;22(2):176–80.
11. Funk M, Richards SB, Desjardins J, et al. Incidence, timing, symptoms, and risk factors for atrial fibrillation after cardiac surgery. Am J Crit Care 2003;12(5): 424–33 [quiz: 434–5].

12. Mozaffarian D, Benjamin EJ, Go AS, et al. Heart disease and stroke statistics-2015 update: a report from the American Heart Association. Circulation 2015; 131(4):e29–322.
13. Steg PG, James SK, Atar D, et al. ESC Guidelines for the management of acute myocardial infarction in patients presenting with ST-segment elevation. Eur Heart J 2012;33(20):2569–619.
14. Body R. Emergent diagnosis of acute coronary syndromes: today's challenges and tomorrow's possibilities. Resuscitation 2008;78(1):13–20.
15. Antman EM, Hand M, Armstrong PW, et al. 2007 focused update of the ACC/AHA 2004 guidelines for the management of patients with ST-Elevation myocardial infarction: a report of the American College of Cardiology/American Heart Association Task Force on Practice Guidelines: developed in collaboration with the Canadian Cardiovascular Society endorsed by the American Academy of Family Physicians: 2007 writing group to review new evidence and update the ACC/AHA 2004 Guidelines for the management of patients with ST-elevation myocardial infarction, writing on behalf of the 2004 writing committee. Circulation 2008; 117(2):296–329.
16. Go AS, Mozaffarian D, Roger VL, et al. Heart disease and stroke statistics–2014 update: a report from the American Heart Association. Circulation 2014;129(3): e28–292.
17. O'Gara PT, Kushner FG, Ascheim DD, et al. 2013 ACCF/AHA guideline for the management of ST-elevation myocardial infarction: a report of the American College of Cardiology Foundation/American Heart Association Task Force on Practice Guidelines. Circulation 2013;127(4):e362–425.
18. Bovino LR, Funk M, Pelter MM, et al. The value of continuous ST-segment monitoring in the emergency department. Adv Emerg Nurs J 2015;37(4):290–300.
19. Bhuiya FA, Pitts SR, McCaig LF. Emergency department visits for chest pain and abdominal pain: United States 1999-2008. NCHS Data Brief 2010;(43):1–8.
20. Kudenchuk PJ, Maynard C, Cobb LA, et al. Utility of the prehospital electrocardiogram in diagnosing acute coronary syndromes: the Myocardial Infarction Triage and Intervention (MITI) Project. J Am Coll Cardiol 1998;32(1):17–27.
21. Zegre-Hemsey J, Sommargren CE, Drew BJ. Initial ECG acquisition within 10 minutes of arrival at the emergency department in persons with chest pain: time and gender differences. J Emerg Nurs 2011;37(1):109–12.
22. Savonitto S, Ardissino D, Granger CB, et al. Prognostic value of the admission electrocardiogram in acute coronary syndromes. JAMA 1999;281(8):707–13.
23. Anderson JL, Adams CD, Antman EM, et al. ACC/AHA 2007 guidelines for the management of patients with unstable angina/non ST-elevation myocardial infarction: a report of the American College of Cardiology/American Heart Association Task Force on Practice Guidelines (Writing Committee to Revise the 2002 Guidelines for the Management of Patients With Unstable Angina/Non ST-Elevation Myocardial Infarction): developed in collaboration with the American College of Emergency Physicians, the Society for Cardiovascular Angiography and Interventions, and the Society of Thoracic Surgeons: endorsed by the American Association of Cardiovascular and Pulmonary Rehabilitation and the Society for Academic Emergency Medicine. Circulation 2007;116(7):e148–304.
24. Bassand JP, Hamm CW, Ardissino D, et al. Guidelines for the diagnosis and treatment of non-ST-segment elevation acute coronary syndromes. Eur Heart J 2007; 28(13):1598–660.

25. Graff L, Palmer AC, Lamonica P, et al. Triage of patients for a rapid (5-minute) electrocardiogram: a rule based on presenting chief complaints. Ann Emerg Med 2000;36(6):554–60.
26. Glickman SW, Shofer FS, Wu MC, et al. Development and validation of a prioritization rule for obtaining an immediate 12-lead electrocardiogram in the emergency department to identify ST-elevation myocardial infarction. Am Heart J 2012;163(3):372–82.
27. Ayer A, Terkelsen CJ. Difficult ECGs in STEMI: lessons learned from serial sampling of pre- and in-hospital ECGs. J Electrocardiol 2014;47(4):448–58.
28. Adams MG, Drew BJ. Body position effects on the ECG: implication for ischemia monitoring. J Electrocardiol 1997;30(4):285–91.
29. Schijvenaars BJ, van Herpen G, Kors JA. Intraindividual variability in electrocardiograms. J Electrocardiol 2008;41(3):190–6.
30. Zegre Hemsey JK, Dracup K, Fleischmann KE, et al. Prehospital electrocardiographic manifestations of acute myocardial ischemia independently predict adverse hospital outcomes. J Emerg Med 2013;44(5):955–61.
31. Zegre Hemsey JK, Dracup K, Fleischmann K, et al. Prehospital 12-lead ST-segment monitoring improves the early diagnosis of acute coronary syndrome. J Electrocardiol 2012;45(3):266–71.
32. Fesmire FM, Percy RF, Bardoner JB, et al. Usefulness of automated serial 12-lead ECG monitoring during the initial emergency department evaluation of patients with chest pain. Ann Emerg Med 1998;31(1):3–11.
33. Fu GY, Joseph AJ, Antalis G. Application of continuous ST-segment monitoring in the detection of silent myocardial ischemia. Ann Emerg Med 1994;23(5):1113–5.
34. Garvey JL, Monk L, Granger CB, et al. Rates of cardiac catheterization cancelation for ST-segment elevation myocardial infarction after activation by emergency medical services or emergency physicians: results from the North Carolina Catheterization Laboratory Activation Registry. Circulation 2012;125(2):308–13.
35. Thygesen K, Alpert JS, Jaffe AS, et al. Third universal definition of myocardial infarction. J Am Coll Cardiol 2012;60(16):1581–98.
36. Drew BJ, Dracup K, Childers R, et al. Finding ECG readers in clinical practice: is it time to change the paradigm? J Am Coll Cardiol 2014;64(5):528.
37. Kushner FG, Hand M, Smith SC Jr, et al. 2009 focused updates: ACC/AHA guidelines for the management of patients with ST-elevation myocardial infarction (updating the 2004 guideline and 2007 focused update) and ACC/AHA/SCAI guidelines on percutaneous coronary intervention (updating the 2005 guideline and 2007 focused update) a report of the American College of Cardiology Foundation/American Heart Association Task Force on Practice Guidelines. J Am Coll Cardiol 2009;54(23):2205–41.
38. Amsterdam EA, Wenger NK, Brindis RG, et al. 2014 AHA/ACC guideline for the management of patients with non-ST-elevation acute coronary syndromes: a report of the American College of Cardiology/American Heart Association Task Force on Practice Guidelines. Circulation 2014;130(25):2354–94.
39. Drew BJ, Krucoff MW. Multilead ST-segment monitoring in patients with acute coronary syndromes: a consensus statement for healthcare professionals. ST-segment monitoring practice guideline International Working Group. Am J Crit Care 1999;8(6):372–86 [quiz: 387–8].
40. Funk M, Winkler CG, May JL, et al. Unnecessary arrhythmia monitoring and underutilization of ischemia and QT interval monitoring in current clinical practice:

baseline results of the Practical Use of the Latest Standards for Electrocardiography trial. J Electrocardiol 2010;43(6):542–7.
41. Patton JA, Funk M. Survey of use of ST-segment monitoring in patients with acute coronary syndromes. Am J Crit Care 2001;10(1):23–32 [quiz: 33–4].
42. Dower GE, Yakush A, Nazzal SB, et al. Deriving the 12-lead electrocardiogram from four (EASI) electrodes. J Electrocardiol 1988;21(Suppl):S182–7.
43. Drew BJ, Adams MG, Pelter MM, et al. ST segment monitoring with a derived 12-lead electrocardiogram is superior to routine cardiac care unit monitoring. Am J Crit Care 1996;5(3):198–206.
44. Drew BJ, Pelter MM, Wung SF, et al. Accuracy of the EASI 12-lead electrocardiogram compared to the standard 12-lead electrocardiogram for diagnosing multiple cardiac abnormalities. J Electrocardiol 1999;32(Suppl):38–47.
45. Pickham D, Drew BJ. QT/QTc interval monitoring in the emergency department. J Emerg Nurs 2008;34(5):428–34.
46. Drew BJ, Ackerman MJ, Funk M, et al. Prevention of torsade de pointes in hospital settings: a scientific statement from the American Heart Association and the American College of Cardiology Foundation. Circulation 2010;121(8):1047–60.

Acute Coronary Syndrome and ST Segment Monitoring

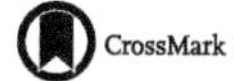

Mary G. Carey, PhD, RN

KEYWORDS

- Coronary artery disease • Myocardial ischemia • Myocardial infarction
- ST segment monitoring • ECG

KEY POINTS

- Three specific conditions are included within acute coronary syndrome: ST elevation myocardial infarction (STEMI), non–ST elevation myocardial infarction (NSTEMI), and unstable angina.
- The ST segment on the electrocardiogram (ECG) is a sensitive and specific marker of myocardial ischemia and infarction.
- STEMIs present as ST elevation whereas NSTEMIs present as ST depression.
- There are no characteristic ECG patterns for unstable angina. What distinguishes unstable angina from STEMI and NSTEMI is that the cardiac biomarkers are not positive for infarction.
- ST segment monitoring can detect silent ischemia, which occurs in the absence of symptoms.

INTRODUCTION

Acute coronary syndrome (ACS) is the second most common cause of hospital emergency department visits in the United States. ACS is caused by a critical obstruction of a coronary artery as a result of atherosclerotic coronary artery disease (CAD).[1] Three specific conditions are included within this syndrome: ST elevation myocardial infarction (STEMI, 30%), non–ST elevation myocardial infarction (NSTEMI, 25%) and unstable angina (38%, **Fig. 1**).[2] Diagnosing myocardial ischemia, a reversible condition before a myocardial infarction (heart attack), is crucial because ischemic heart disease increases the risk of death among the survivors. Approximately 1.5 million Americans will have a heart attack this year as a result of myocardial ischemia and nearly 30% of

The author has nothing to disclose.

Clinical Nursing Research Center, Strong Memorial Hospital, University of Rochester Medical Center, University of Rochester School of Nursing, 601 Elmwood Avenue, Box 619-7, Rochester, NY 14642, USA
E-mail address: mary_carey@urmc.rochester.edu

Crit Care Nurs Clin N Am 28 (2016) 347–355
http://dx.doi.org/10.1016/j.cnc.2016.04.006 ccnursing.theclinics.com
0899-5885/16/$ – see front matter © 2016 Elsevier Inc. All rights reserved.

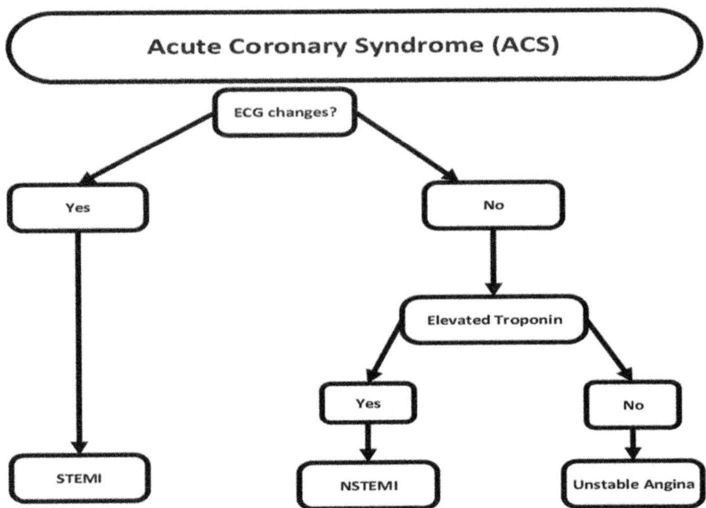

Fig. 1. ACS flow diagram.

them will be fatal.[1] Importantly, treating ACS has tremendous benefits because both coronary artery revascularization and pharmacologic therapies significantly reduce morbidity and mortality.[3] Because ACS is prevalent and deadly, yet treatable, early diagnosis is vital. The diagnosis of ACS can be difficult to make because the symptoms are not reliable and range from no symptoms (asymptomatic) to crushing chest pain. Frequently, the disease is diagnosed only after the patient has had a heart attack. Given that CAD is part of normal aging, the disease occurs in the young and the old, in women and men, and in patients with and patients without comorbidities.

Historically, hospital cardiac monitoring was for the detection of heart rate and then evolved to detecting obvious ventricular cardiac arrhythmias (ventricular tachycardia). Over the years, cardiac monitoring has become more sophisticated, also recording nonlethal atrial arrhythmias (atrial fibrillation). Currently, lethal arrhythmias sound a level 1 alarm, resulting in a high-pitched siren demanding everyone's attention, which, by law, may not be disabled.

More recently, researchers discovered that the ST segment on the electrocardiogram (ECG) is a sensitive and specific marker of myocardial ischemia and infarction. Thus, a new purpose for in-hospital cardiac monitoring emerged called ST segment monitoring. This article describes ACS and infarction and the application of ST segment monitoring in detecting these conditions.

MYOCARDIAL INFARCTION

ST Elevation Myocardial Infarction

Untreated myocardial ischemia (injury) leads to myocardial infarction (death). Once cardiac cells die, proteins are released and detected in blood tests, verifying that a myocardial infarction (heart attack has occurred). In addition to the blood test, ECG changes accompany a myocardial infarction, representing myocardial cell death and the inability of the cell to contract; often, later, represented by a Q wave.

One of the 2 types of myocardial infarction seen in patients with ACS is supply-related ischemia, which results from complete coronary artery occlusion. Coronary artery occlusion is brought on by the disruption of atherosclerotic plaque followed by cycles of plaque rupture, coronary vasospasm, platelet stimulation, and thrombus formation with resultant loss of blood flow.[4–6] Because this type of ischemia threatens the entire thickness (transmural) of the myocardial wall, immediate treatment to reestablish blood flow to the heart is essential (**Fig. 2**).

Electrocardiographic Patterns

The typical ECG manifestation of total supply-related ischemia is ST segment elevation visible in the ECG leads that lie directly over the ischemic myocardial zone. The third universal definition of myocardial infarction[7] was developed by the members of professional societies of the American College of Cardiology and the American Heart Association to increase the sensitivity and specificity of the ECG by recognizing age, sex, and ECG lead differences. In the absence of left ventricular hypertrophy and left bundle branch block, the ECG criteria include

- New ST elevation at the J-point in 2 contiguous leads with the cut-points: greater than or equal to 0.2 mV in men 40 years or older; greater than or equal to 0.25 mV in men younger than 40 years, or greater than or equal to 0.15 mV in women in leads V_2 to V_3 and/or greater than or equal to 0.1 mV in all other leads (**Fig. 3**).
- New ST depression and T-wave changes defined by new horizontal or down-sloping ST depression greater than or equal to 0.05 mV in 2 contiguous leads and/or T inversion greater than or equal to 0.1 mV in 2 contiguous leads with prominent R wave or R/S ratio greater than 1.

However, a year later, in 2013, the American College of Cardiology and the American Heart Association simplified these recommendations in their STEMI guidelines. In these guidelines, the ST segment elevation threshold was measured at the J point in 2 contiguous leads or more of 0.2 mV or more in men or 0.15 mV or more in women in leads V2 and V3 and/or of 0.1 mV or more in all other leads.[8] More than just the quantification of the ST segment, the value is in trending a change over time. In non-ACS patients, the ST segment remains fixed throughout the hospitalization; however, among ACS patients, an ST segment shift may indicate an acute change in the patient's cardiac condition.

Regional, Not Global

Unlike arrhythmias, which affect the heart globally, STEMI ECG patterns are regional. For example, if a patient is suffering from ventricular tachycardia, any of the ECG leads

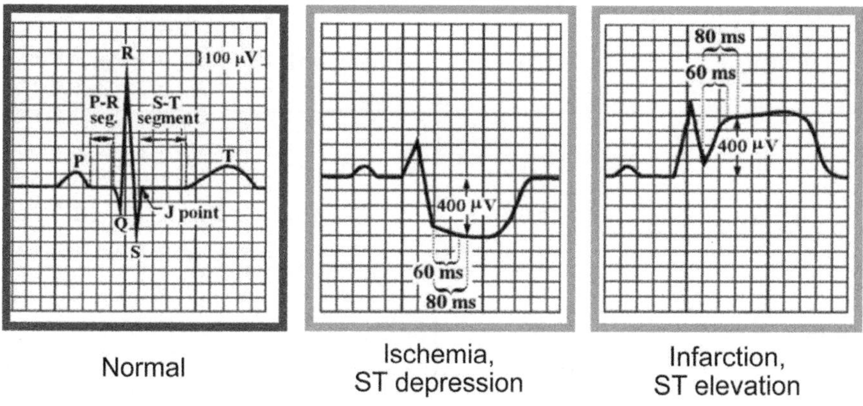

Fig. 2. ECG characteristics of ischemia and infarction and representation of the injury on the left ventricular wall.

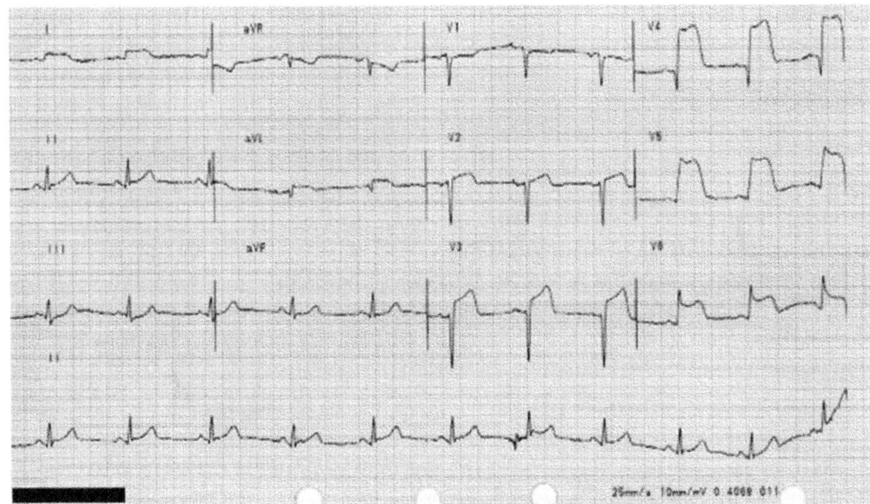

Fig. 3. Resting 12-lead ECG. Sinus rhythm at 70 beats per minute with an acute septal (V2) anterior (V3 and V4) lateral (V5, V6, I, aVL) myocardial infarction with an ST elevation. Note the 2 most commonly monitored leads, VI and II, do not have ST segment deviation so this acute infarct would not be detected by clinicians.

will display the characteristically rapid organized lethal rhythm. However, with infarction, the ECG leads need to be placed over the affected area to capture the ST segment deviation (**Fig. 4**). The 4 anatomic groups include septal (V1 and V2), anterior (V3 and V4), lateral (V5, V6, I, and aVL) and inferior (II, III, and aVF).

So, occlusion of the right coronary artery typically produces ST segment elevation in leads II, III, and aVF. Occlusion of the left anterior descending coronary artery typically produces ST segment elevation in leads V2, V3, and V4; however, identification of total coronary occlusion of the left circumflex coronary artery (LCX) is more complex because placement of the standard ECG electrodes is on the anterior chest, which

I Lateral	aVR None	V_1 Septal	V_4 Anterior
II Inferior	aVL Lateral	V_2 Septal	V_5 Lateral
III Inferior	aVF Inferior	V_3 Anterior	V_6 Lateral

Fig. 4. Anatomic groups of the resting 12-lead ECG.

is opposite of the heart wall that is supplied by the LCX. So, occlusion of the LCX may produce ST segment depression in leads V1, V2, or V3, which reflects the reciprocal, or mirror image, ST segment elevation occurring in the posterior wall of the left ventricle, whereas in some patients ST segment changes may also be seen in leads I and aVL.[9]

Non–ST Elevation Myocardial Infarction

A second type of ischemia for which patients with ACS or stable angina are at risk is demand-related ischemia. This type of ischemia occurs when the demand for oxygen exceeds the flow capabilities of a coronary artery (exercise, tachycardia, or stress). Patients with this type of ischemia are likely to have stable atherosclerotic plaque. The ST segment pattern of demand-related ischemia is ST segment depression, often appearing in several ECG leads (**Fig. 5**).

UNSTABLE ANGINA

Unstable angina is an acceleration of stable angina that does not spontaneously resolve; ECG changes may or may not occur. Unstable angina does not result in myocardial death, thus there is no elevation in the cardiac biomarkers indicating infarction. Unstable angina is caused by myocardial ischemia, the condition in which there is an inadequate supply of blood to the heart. At this stage, it is a reversible condition because the coronary artery is not blocked but rather the lumen of the coronary is compromised, resulting in a diminished blood supply. If myocardial ischemia continues, it leads to myocardial infarction or cell death (heart attack), which is not reversible.

Electrocardiographic Patterns

There are no characteristic patterns of ECGs for unstable angina. What distinguishes unstable angina from STEMI and NSTEMI is that the cardiac biomarkers are not positive for infarction.

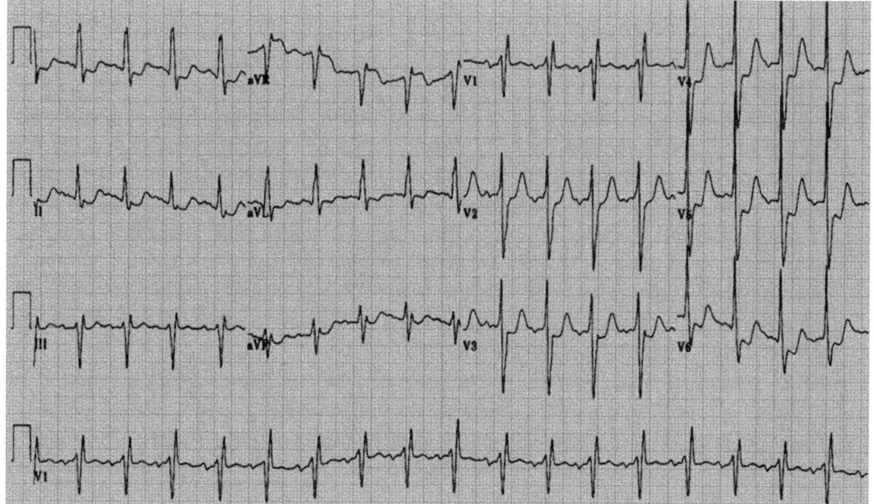

Fig. 5. Resting 12-lead ECG. Sinus tachycardia at 150 beats per minute with anterior lateral ST segment depression. The coronaries are unable to meet the demand of the heart rate, thus immediate efforts should be made to reduce the heart rate.

ST SEGMENT MONITORING

Bedside ST segment monitoring provides ongoing surveillance for detection of transient myocardial ischemia. This technology should be applied to patients who are being evaluated or are diagnosed with ACS, including unstable angina and acute myocardial infarction. For these patients, continuous ST segment monitoring is valuable in detecting recurrent or transient ischemia and in determining the success of thrombolytic therapy and percutaneous coronary intervention (PCI).

Ideally, diagnosis of ACS should be done with continuous monitoring of all 12 ECG leads because the mechanism of ACS varies. The occlusive coronary type (ruptured coronary plaque) yields distinct ST segment elevation whereas the demand-related type (not enough coronary supply to meet demand) results in ST segment depression in specific ECG leads. If only 2 ECG leads are available, however, the best 2 for ischemia detection are leads III and V3.[10] Patient-specific monitoring also may be done if a prior 12-lead ECG was obtained during acute ischemia (STEMI, PCI, or treadmill testing). In this scenario, the ECG leads showing maximal ST segment deviation should be selected for continuous monitoring to detect recurrent ischemia.

Asymptomatic Myocardial Ischemia and Infarction

Continuous monitoring of the ECG for ischemic ST segment changes is more reliable than patient symptoms because more than three-quarters of ECG-detected ischemic events occur without patient symptoms.[6,10–13] Patients who have transient ischemia detected with continuous ST segment monitoring are more likely to have unfavorable outcomes, including myocardial infarction and death, compared with patients without such events.[6,10–16] Given the dynamic, unpredictable, and silent nature of ACS, continuous ECG monitoring of patients for ischemia is essential.[17] Importantly, ST segment monitoring can detect silent ischemia, which occurs in the absence of symptoms.

Indications

According to current consensus statements,[10,18] multilead ST segment monitoring is indicated in most patients with the following diagnoses:

- In the early phase of ACS (STEMI, NSTEMI, and unstable angina) patients should be monitored for a minimum of 24 hours or until they remain event-free for 12 to 24 hours.
- Patients with chest pain (or the anginal equivalent, heartburn) that prompts a visit to the emergency department should undergo ST segment monitoring for 8 to 12 hours in combination with testing serum cardiac biomarkers for infarction, which may be a cost-effective way to triage patients who arrive at the emergency department with chest pain. Given the transient nature of ST segment changes, serial resting 12-lead ECG should be obtained every 15 to 30 minutes in patients with ongoing symptoms in whom the initial ECG is not diagnostic of a STEMI.[7] This is especially true in the elderly, women, and diabetic patients who frequently present with atypical symptoms of ACS.[19]
- After nonurgent PCI procedures with suboptimal results, monitoring should be initiated immediately postprocedure and continue for 24 hours or longer if arrhythmias or ST segment deviation events occur. According to these same guidelines,[10,18] ST segment monitoring may be of benefit for the following cases:
  - Postacute myocardial infarction
  - After nonurgent uncomplicated PCI
  - Patients at high risk for ischemia after cardiac or noncardiac surgery
  - Variant angina resulting from coronary vasospasm.

ST segment monitoring may not be appropriate for certain patient groups because current software cannot reliably interpret ST segment changes resulting from myocardial ischemia and leads to false-positive alarms, contributing to alarm fatigue.[6,10,18] Specifically, it may not be suitable to monitor patients with the following:

- Left bundle-branch block
- Ventricular paced rhythm
- Confounding dysrhythmias that obscure the ST segment
- Agitation causing excessive artifact.

Reducing False-Positive Alarms

Application of the ECG electrodes is often done with little care. Clinicians may just ask patients to pull their shift up and slap the adhesive stickers to the chest wall, which will generate an ECG waveform but not necessarily a correct waveform. Ideally, the clinician should place the patient in a resting supine position in bed and expose the patient's torso while maintaining modesty. This preparation provides access to the patient's chest for accurate electrode placement and ensures that an artifact-free ECG is obtained. Experts recommend marking the locations of the chest electrodes (precordial leads) with indelible ink to assure that when electrodes are removed they can be replaced in their original locations. For example, V2 and V3 are removed to view the pericardial window for an echocardiogram. Precordial electrodes are extremely sensitive to placement so that if they are incorrectly placed as little as 1 cm away from their original location the waveforms on the ECG change.[20,21]

Accurate ECG monitoring assures that clinicians note and interpret ST segment changes for timely detection of myocardial ischemia. There may be an increase in the number of bedside alarms when the ST segment software is initiated, which may be caused by actual ischemia, body-position changes, transient dysrhythmias, heart rate changes, artifacts, or lead misplacement.[22] Nonischemic ST segment changes can occur and should be considered when evaluating ST segment trend changes, including movement of the skin electrodes, dysrhythmias, intermittent bundle-branch block pattern, body position changes, and ventricular paced rhythms.[10,22,23]

SUMMARY

Technology has evolved and cardiac monitors have became smaller, portable, and affordable, so it is now estimated that nearly 80% of hospitalized beds have cardiac monitoring. Thus, a variety of bedside and telemetry cardiac monitors are currently available for use in clinical practice. Most, if not all, are equipped with ST segment monitoring software; however, clinicians must proactively activate the software and set patient-specific parameters. Overtime, clinicians should monitor the trend of the ST segments and evaluate any ST segment change (elevation or depression) for possible myocardial ischemia.[24] Importantly, patient symptoms are not a reliable way to detect myocardial ischemia or infarction whereas ST segment monitoring can detect silent ischemia that occurs in the absence of symptoms.

REFERENCES

1. Mozaffarian D, Benjamin EJ, Go AS, et al, American Heart Association Statistics Committee and Stroke Statistics Subcommittee. Heart disease and stroke statistics—2015 update: a report from the American Heart Association. Circulation 2015;131(4):e29–322.

2. Torres M, Moayedi S. Evaluation of the acutely dyspneic elderly patient. Clin Geriatr Med 2007;23(2):307–25.
3. Morrison LJ, Neumar RW, Zimmerman JL, et al. Strategies for improving survival after in-hospital cardiac arrest in the United States: 2013 consensus recommendations: a consensus statement from the American Heart Association. Circulation 2013;127(14):1538–63.
4. Cura FA, Escudero AG, Berrocal D, et al. Protection of distal embolization in high-risk patients with acute ST-segment elevation myocardial infarction (PREMIAR). Am J Cardiol 2007;99(3):357–63.
5. DeWood MA, Spores J, Notske R, et al. Prevalence of total coronary occlusion during the early hours of transmural myocardial infarction. N Engl J Med 1980; 303(16):897–902.
6. Gottlieb SO, Weisfeldt ML, Ouyang P, et al. Silent ischemia as a marker for early unfavorable outcomes in patients with unstable angina. N Engl J Med 1986; 314(19):1214–9.
7. Thygesen K, Alpert JS, Jaffe AS, et al. Third universal definition of myocardial infarction. Circulation 2012;126(16):2020–35.
8. O'Gara PT, Kushner FG, Ascheim DD, et al. 2013 ACCF/AHA guideline for the management of ST-elevation myocardial infarction: a report of the American College of Cardiology Foundation/American Heart Association Task Force on Practice Guidelines. J Am Coll Cardiol 2013;61(4):e78–140.
9. Stephens KE, Anderson H, Carey MG, et al. Interpreting 12-lead electrocardiograms for acute ST-Elevation myocardial infarction: what nurses know. J Cardiovasc Nurs 2007;22(3):186–93.
10. Drew BJC, Robert M, Funk M, et al. AHA scientific statement: practice standards for electrocardiographic monitoring in hospital settings: an American Heart Association scientific statement from the councils on cardiovascular nursing, clinical cardiology, and cardiovascular disease in the young: endorsed by the international society of computerized electrocardiology and the American Association of Critical-Care Nurses. J Cardiovasc Nurs 2005;20(2):76–106.
11. Adams MG, Pelter MM, Wung S-F, et al. Frequency of silent myocardial ischemia with 12-lead ST segment monitoring in the coronary care unit: are there sex-related differences? Heart Lung 1999;28(2):81–6.
12. Drew BJ, Harris P, Zègre-Hemsey JK, et al. Insights into the problem of alarm fatigue with physiologic monitor devices: a comprehensive observational study of consecutive intensive care unit patients. PLoS One 2014;9(10):e110274.
13. Pelter MM, Adams MG, Drew BJ. Transient myocardial ischemia is an independent predictor of adverse in-hospital outcomes in patients with acute coronary syndromes treated in the telemetry unit. Heart Lung 2003;32(2):71–8.
14. Akkerhuis KM, Klootwijk PAJ, Lindeboom W, et al. Recurrent ischaemia during continuous multilead ST-segment monitoring identifies patients with acute coronary syndromes at high risk of adverse cardiac events; meta-analysis of three studies involving 995 patients. Eur Heart J 2001;22(21):1997–2006.
15. Drew BJ, Pelter MM, Adams MG. Frequency, characteristics, and clinical significance of transient ST segment elevation in patients with acute coronary syndromes. Eur Heart J 2002;23(12):941–7.
16. Drew BJ, Pelter MM, Lee E, et al. Designing prehospital ECG systems for acute coronary syndromes. Lessons learned from clinical trials involving 12-lead ST-segment monitoring. J Electrocardiol 2005;38(4 Suppl):180–5.
17. Krucoff MW, Croll MA, Pope JE, et al. Continuously updated 12-lead ST-segment recovery analysis for myocardial infarct artery patency assessment and its

correlation with multiple simultaneous early angiographic observations. Am J Cardiol 1993;71(2):145–51.

18. Drew BJ, Krucoff MW. Multilead ST-segment monitoring in patients with acute coronary syndromes: a consensus statement for healthcare professionals. ST-Segment Monitoring Practice Guideline International Working Group. Am J Crit Care 1999;8(6):372–86.
19. Canto JG, Shlipak MG, Rogers WJ, et al. PRevalence, clinical characteristics, and mortality among patients with myocardial infarction presenting without chest pain. JAMA 2000;283(24):3223–9.
20. Drew BJ, Califf RM, Funk M, et al. Practice standards for electrocardiographic monitoring in hospital settings: an American Heart Association scientific statement from the Councils on Cardiovascular Nursing, Clinical Cardiology, and Cardiovascular Disease in the Young: endorsed by the International Society of Computerized electrocardiology and the American Association of Critical-Care Nurses. Circulation 2004;110(17):2721–46.
21. Wenger W, Kligfield P. Variability of precordial electrode placement during routine electrocardiography. J Electrocardiol 1996;29(3):179–84.
22. Drew BJ, Wung SF, Adams MG, et al. Bedside diagnosis of myocardial ischemia with ST-segment monitoring technology: measurement issues for real-time clinical decision making and trial designs. J Electrocardiol 1998;30(Suppl):157–65.
23. Adams M, Drew BJ. Body position effects on the ECG: implication for ischemia monitoring. J Electrocardiol 1997;30(4):285–91.
24. Pelter MM, Kozik TM, Loranger DL, et al. A research method for detecting transient myocardial ischemia in patients with suspected acute coronary syndrome using continuous ST-segment analysis. J Vis Exp 2012;(70):50124.

Basic Cardiac Electrophysiology and Common Drug-induced Arrhythmias

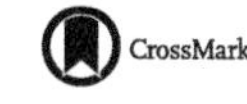

Aimee Lee, CNS, ACNP-BC[a,1], David Pickham, RN, PhD[b,*]

KEYWORDS

- Drug-induced • Arrhythmias • Electrocardiography • Automaticity
- Triggered activity • Re-entry • Proarrhythmic

KEY POINTS

- Cardiac function is dependent on normal electrical and mechanical activity.
- Many drugs administered to alleviate symptoms also have the negative side effect of altering cardiac function.
- At the cellular level, drugs often block or interact with ion channel functioning and most commonly impact cardiac repolarization.
- Triggered activity, automaticity, and re-entry are 3 typical mechanisms for drug-induced arrhythmia.
- Understanding cell activity and action potentials helps in understanding how drugs can interact and cause arrhythmias.

INTRODUCTION

Drugs can be a double-edged sword, providing the benefit of symptom alleviation and disease modification, but potentially causing harm from adverse cardiac arrhythmic events. Drug-induced arrhythmias are defined as the production of de novo arrhythmias or aggravation of existing arrhythmias as a result of previous or concomitant pharmacologic treatment.[1] Drug-induced arrhythmia episodes were first described in patients receiving quinidine,[2] an antiarrhythmic, and within the last few years a variety of cardiovascular and noncardiovascular drugs have been shown to possess proarrhythmic properties. These properties arise from several electrophysiologically distinct and identifiable mechanisms,[3] the most common of which impairs cardiac

Disclosure Statement: The authors have nothing to disclose.

[a] Cardiac Electrophysiology, Stanford Health Care, 300 Pasteur Drive, Stanford, CA 94305, USA;
[b] General Medical Disciplines, Stanford Medicine, Stanford, CA, USA
[1] Present address: c/o Suite I238, 301 Ravenswood Avenue, Menlo Park, CA 94025.
* Corresponding author. c/o Suite I238, 301 Ravenswood Avenue, Menlo Park, CA 94025.
E-mail address: dpickham@stanfordhealthcare.org

Crit Care Nurs Clin N Am 28 (2016) 357–371
http://dx.doi.org/10.1016/j.cnc.2016.04.007 ccnursing.theclinics.com
0899-5885/16/$ – see front matter © 2016 Elsevier Inc. All rights reserved.

repolarization.[4] The purpose of this review is to summarize normal cardiac cell and tissue function, to look at the actions of common drugs that affect cardiac repolarization, and to examine the adverse effects of commonly administered antiarrhythmics.

CARDIAC ACTION POTENTIAL

At an organ level, normal electrical activation of the heart begins in the sinus node, initiating an ongoing activation of atrial muscle cells and continuing to the atrioventricular (AV) node. The AV node delays the activation toward the ventricles, optimizing the time for filling of the ventricles by the atrial contraction. In the ventricles, the AV node is connected to the His-Purkinje system. The His-Purkinje system acts as a fast "highway" distributing the electrical activation in the ventricles toward the ventricular myocardial cells. The specialized cells forming this conduction system are known as pacemaker cells (sinus nodal, AV nodal, and His-Purkinje cells), and the contractile units within the heart are known as myocardial cells (atrial and ventricular).

All myocardial cells possess 2 inherent characteristics that can contribute to arrhythmias: conductivity (the ability to transmit an electrical impulse) and excitability (the ability to respond to an electrical impulse). Pacemaker cells also possess an extra characteristic that can cause arrhythmias, automaticity: the ability to spontaneously generate electrical impulses. Central to the ability to perform any of these functions is the cells action potential (AP) (**Fig. 1**). The AP is an elegant interplay of multiple types of ions moving over the myocardial cell membrane. Regulating most ion movements are special types of transmembrane proteins called voltage-gated ion channels. These ion channels span across the cell membrane and provide a mechanism, much like a doorway, for the movement of ions into and outside the cell. Review of cellular cardiac depolarization and repolarization illustrates the function of these ion channels.

When a stimulus reaches a resting myocardial cell, alterations in the membrane's potential triggers specific voltage-gated sodium channels to open. Opening these channels allows sodium to rush into the cell, resulting in cardiac depolarization, and is considered phase 0 of the AP. In phase 1 of the AP, the increase in membrane potential peaks, triggering the closure of the sodium voltage-gated channels and the

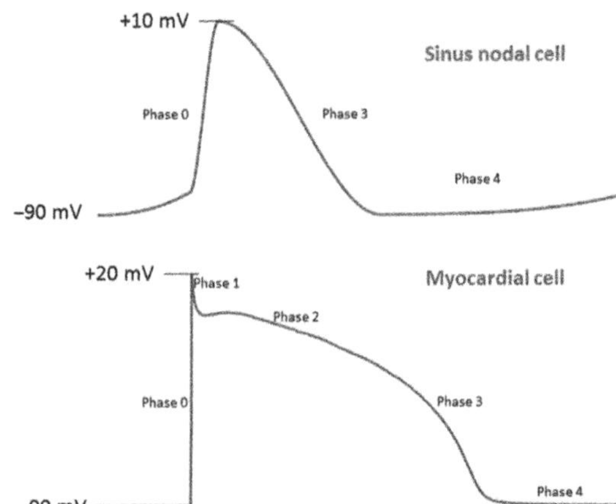

Fig. 1. Myocardial and pacemaker APs. The pacemaker cells do not express phases 1 and 2 of the typical AP of myocardial cells and never truly reach a "resting state." (*Courtesy of* Peter van Dam, PhD, PEACS BV, Arnhem, Netherlands.)

opening of multiple outward potassium channels. This process allows potassium to extrude from the cell into the extracellular space and causes a sudden drop in the cells' membrane potential; this is the beginning of cardiac repolarization. A distinctive plateau phase indicates phase 2 of the AP and is the result of a balance between inward calcium and outward potassium ions. During this phase, a high concentration of intracellular calcium contributes to a cascade of actions resulting in a mechanical contraction of the cell. As the calcium channels close, phase 3 of the AP begins. This phase is known as late repolarization and is the phase before the cell is fully repolarized. During phase 3, outward flow of potassium ions continues to dominate, driving the resting potential of the cell below threshold, typically less than −70 mV, and into the fourth and final phase. Phase 4 is known as the "resting state." Here, the membrane potential is stable and in a state that is able to be responsive to any new external stimulus.

It is important to note that different cell types have unique AP characteristics that are important for normal cardiac functioning. Pacemaker cell activity, for example, is dependent on slow inward calcium currents and not the fast sodium currents that are responsible for depolarizing myocardial cells. Unlike myocardial cells, pacemaker cells never truly reach a "resting state" and are always active. After repolarizing, the transmembrane potential gradually and spontaneously begins to depolarize again; this continual rhythmic action is the mechanism underpinning the cardiac rate.

INTRINSIC MECHANISMS OF ARRHYTHMIA

There are both intrinsic and extrinsic mechanisms of arrhythmias. Understanding the normal AP is important in determining the different mechanisms for arrhythmia. There are 3 main intrinsic mechanisms for cardiac arrhythmias: abnormal automaticity, triggered activity (TA), and re-entry. Identifying the specific mechanism can be challenging; however, differentiating and understanding the underlying mechanism for arrhythmia are critical to the development of an appropriate diagnosis and treatment strategy. The following is a description of these mechanisms (**Fig. 2**).

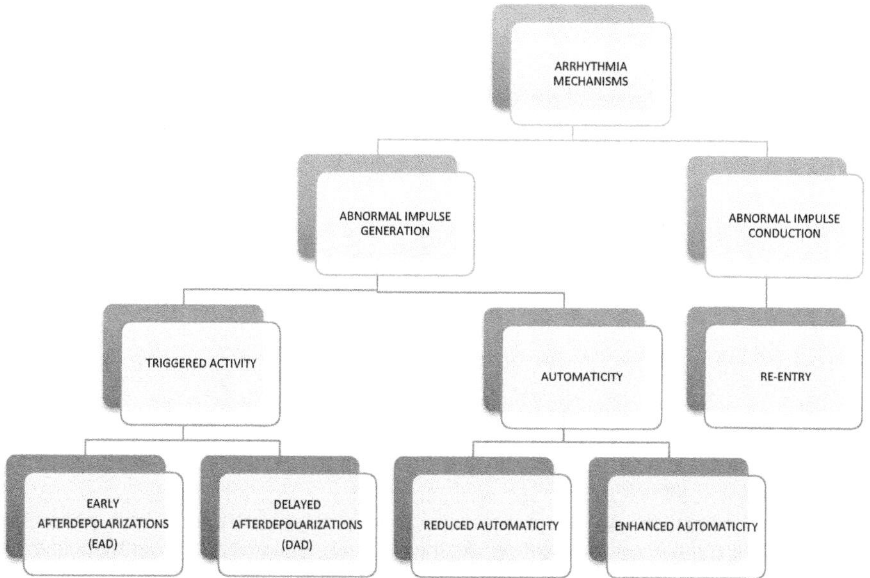

Fig. 2. Mechanisms of cardiac arrhythmia.

Abnormal Automaticity

Pacemaker cells have an inherent ability to spontaneously reach threshold potential and depolarize. The time it takes for the pacemaker cell to perform this function, the action potential duration (APD), is dependent on the cell's location within the heart. For instance, the APD of the sinoatrial (SA) node is much shorter than that of both the AV node and the Purkinje fibers. Therefore, because of this inherent speed, the SA node acts as the predominate pacemaker, controlling the cardiac rate and rhythm. When the SA node fails to function as the primary pacemaker, arrhythmias occur. Arrhythmias may occur when an ectopic cell outside the SA node generates and propagates an electrical impulse that overrides and usurps control from the SA node, or with SA node dysfunction. In a heart with a diseased SA node, control is quickly re-established by another group of pacemaker cells extrinsic to the SA node.

Triggered Activity

TA results when an impulse causes depolarization of the myocardial cell before repolarization has been fully completed. These types of errant depolarizations are called afterdepolarizations and can occur early during phase 2 of the AP (early afterdepolarizations [EAD]) or later during phase 3 of the AP (delayed afterdepolarization [DAD]) (**Fig. 3**). Depending on the strength of the afterdepolarization, an impulse may cross the threshold potential triggering the cell to fully depolarize, and if adjacent cells are near threshold, propagate to cause arrhythmia. Factors that may contribute to the heart's susceptibility for developing afterdepolarizations are electrolyte abnormalities, acidosis, hypoxemia, and an increased catecholamine state.

Re-entry

With normal cardiac activity, a depolarization wave front is initiated within the SA node and travels through specialized conduction pathways in an organized sequence throughout the heart. This wave front terminates when the activating wave hits cells that are refractory and thus are unable to propagate the activation. In re-entry, the original impulse continues to be propagated by an aberrant pathway, as a result of

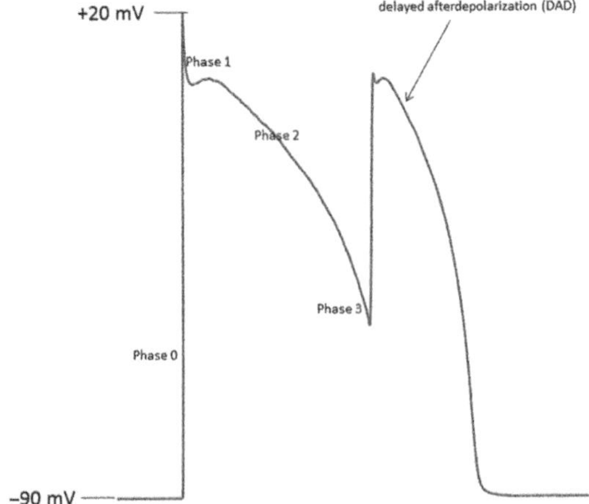

Fig. 3. Triggered activity. An external stimulus triggered depolarization within phase 3 of the AP, before complete repolarization. As the cell had repolarized sufficiently below the threshold potential, a rogue depolarization was triggered. (*Courtesy of* Peter van Dam, PhD, PEACS BV, Arnhem, Netherlands.)

disease, such as myocardial infarction, or refractory, because of recent depolarization (or both) (**Fig. 4**). A path of slowed conduction allows sufficient recovery of the refractory cells behind the propagating wave front, resulting in continued propagation of the activation (**Fig. 5**). Common causes for re-entry arrhythmias are as follows:

- Structural heart disease: slow conduction and abnormal scar-based heterogeneous conduction delays[5]
- Dual pathway AV nodal tissue: 2 physiologically distinct AV nodal cells types: one with fast action and longer refractory periods, and the other with slower action and shorter refractory periods,[6] can result in AV nodal re-entry tachycardia (AVNRT)
- Wolff-Parkinson-White syndrome (WPW)[7]: a congenital anomaly of conductive cardiac tissue bridging the atrium and the ventricle; this can cause AV re-entry tachycardia

EXTRINSIC MECHANISMS OF ARRHYTHMIA

The extrinsic mechanisms of arrhythmia are acquired long QT syndrome (LQTS) and acquired short QT syndrome (SQTS). Modern medicine is predicated on the effective identification of drug targets and development of drugs targets that are aimed at alleviating or curing disease. However, not all drug effects are beneficial. The alteration of cardiac repolarization has been shown to be one of the most common adverse effects of both cardiac and noncardiac drugs[8]; this is known as acquired LQTS.

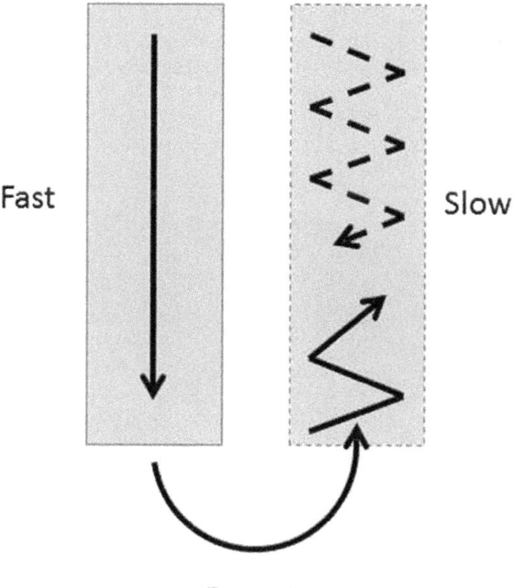

Fig. 4. Re-entry activity. Activation moves rapidly down the "Fast" pathway, reaching the end before complete depolarization of the "Slow" pathway. As the cells within the lower portion of the "Slow" pathway are in a state waiting to be activated, the activation from the "Fast" pathway can be propagated in a retrograde direction up the "Slow" pathway. This is the basis for the arrhythmia, AVNRT.

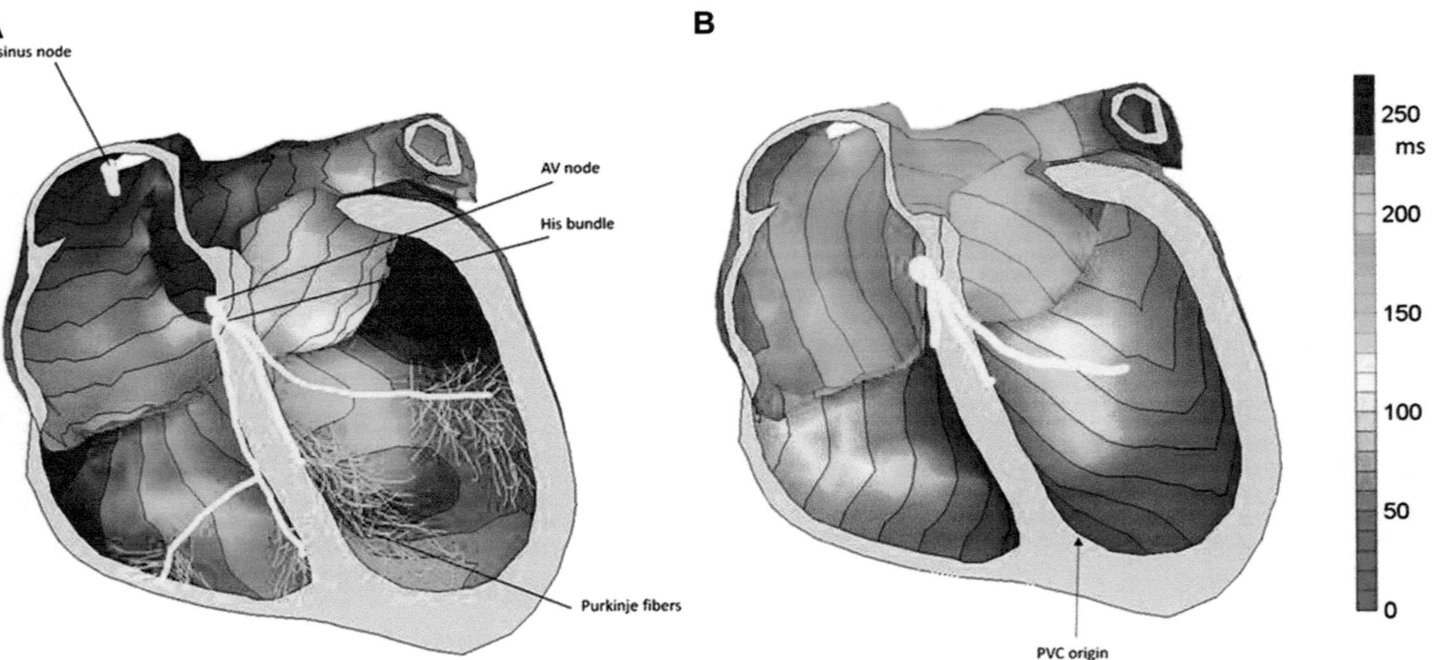

Fig. 5. (*A*) Isochron diagram of normal cardiac conduction. The figure shows the timing of activation throughout the heart. The SA node initiates depolarization and is shown in red, corresponding with time zero. Over the next 120 milliseconds, the atria activate. After a short delay in the AV node, the activation wave front moves throughout the ventricles, depolarizing these tissues 200 milliseconds after initiation from the SA node. (*B*) Isochron of abnormal action cardiac conduction. In the same heart, activation is now shown from an ectopic site: left ventricular septum. This activation has retrograde conduction to the atria from the AV node. Consequently, the atrial activation ends in the left auricle. (*Courtesy of* Peter van Dam, PhD, PEACS BV, Arnhem, Netherlands.)

Acquired Long QT Syndrome

LQTS is a congenital disorder that can cause torsades de pointes (TdP), syncope, and death. TdP refers to a polymorphic ventricular tachycardia that occurs in the setting of an abnormally prolonged QT interval. In the acquired form of LQTS, multiple risk factors have been associated with QT prolongation, but the use of proarrhythmic drugs is the most common.[9,10] These drugs have been shown to directly interact or indirectly act on potassium voltage-gated ion channels, physically blocking the ability of potassium to extrude from the cell, resulting in prolongation of both phase 2 and phase 3 of ventricular repolarization. Many drugs and drug classes have been identified as contributors to LQTS (**Table 1**).

Clinical features

Acquired LQTS is identified by prolongation of the QT interval and is currently defined as a rate-corrected QT interval greater than 470 ms for men and 480 ms for women.[11] Patients with a change of more than 60 ms from baseline after receiving a known QT interval (repolarization) prolonging drug are also at high risk for arrhythmia.[12] The electrocardiographic features of TdP are distinctive and are described as a "twisting of the points" on the electrocardiogram (ECG).[13] Although distinctive, TdP is only truly distinguishable from ventricular fibrillation by analyzing the few beats immediately preceding the arrhythmia. TdP is known to have a pause-dependent onset, a short-long-short sequence before arrhythmia (**Fig. 6**), which is typically absent with ventricular fibrillation.[3]

Treatment

After correctly identifying the arrhythmia, it is important to withdraw all known QT prolonging drugs and correct for any electrolyte disturbances (class I, level of evidence: A).[11] To reduce the susceptibility for further TA, administration of magnesium, an essential transmembranous and intracellular myocardial cell modulator, should be considered. An intravenous bolus of 2 g of magnesium sulfate followed by a second

Table 1
Common Long QT drug classes

Drug Group	Drugs
Antiarrhythmic	Disopyramide, procainamide, quinidine, mexiletine, D,L-sotalol
Antineoplastic	Tamoxifen
Antifungal	Itraconazole, ketoconazole, fluconazole, voriconazole
Antimicrobial	Erythromycin, clarithromycin, azithromycin, levofloxacin, moxifloxacin, ofloxacin, trimethoprim-sulfamethoxazole, pentamidine, quinine, chloroquine
Antihistamine	Diphenhydramine, hydroxyzine
Antidepressant	Venlafaxine, fluoxetine, desipramine, imipramine, paroxetine, sertraline, citalopram, escitalopram
Antipsychotic	Chlorpromazine, prochlorperazine, haloperidol, droperidol, risperidone, chloral hydrate
Antimigraine	Naratriptan, sumatriptan, zolmitriptan
Diuretics	Indapamide, thiazide, furosemide
Gastrointestinal stimulants	Cisapride, metoclopramide, domperidone
Hormones	Octreotide, vasopressin

Full lists of drugs associated with QT prolongation are available at: https://www.crediblemeds.org/.

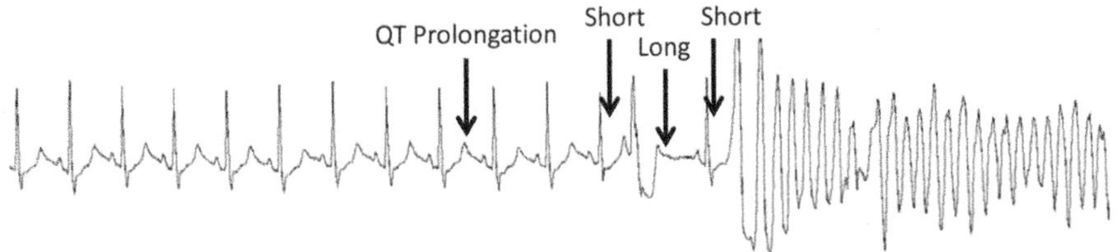

Fig. 6. ECG Example of TdP. In this example, note the prolongation of the QT interval before the arrhythmia initiation, short-long-short complexes; this differentiates TdP from other polymorphic ventricular tachycardias or ventricular fibrillation. (*Courtesy of* Eric Helfenbein, Philips Healthcare, San Jose, California.)

bolus is effective in terminating most episodes of TdP.[14] If profound bradycardia is present, cardiac pacing is indicated. Cardiac pacing will increase the heart rate and eliminate long pauses that may enable the substrate to develop TA, and thus, consequently, ventricular tachycardia. Alternatively, administration of isoproterenol, a drug that stimulates β-receptors in the heart, may also be used to increase the heart rate, although this should only be used when transvenous pacing cannot be immediately implemented.[15]

Acquired Short QT Syndrome

SQTS is a newly identified and rare congenital abnormality that is characterized by significant shortening of repolarization time.[16] It is thought that reduced repolarization time promotes TA and provides conditions for re-entry.[17] The most common drug known to shorten the QT interval is digoxin. Digoxin is intended to act by inhibiting cellular sodium-potassium exchange pumps, which in turn reverses sodium-calcium exchange pumps, resulting in increased intracellular calcium and sodium overload.[12] Because of its actions, almost all arrhythmias, besides atrial fibrillation and atrial flutter, have been associated with its toxicity.[18] The intracellular calcium overload, coupled with digoxin's vagotonic action, promotes abnormal automaticity and DADs.[19] Other conditions that can contribute to the acquired form of SQTS are electrolyte imbalances, acidosis, hyperthermia, and increased catecholamines.[17] Importantly, the lone presence of a shorter-than-normal QT interval is insufficient to be diagnostic for the congenital form of SQTS. Proarrhythmia with shorter-than-normal QT intervals, unlike acquired QT interval prolongation, is rare.[20]

Clinical features

The distinguishing feature of this abnormality is a shortened QT interval on the ECG. Consensus is lacking as to the true diagnostic risk threshold for SQTS; however, recent guidelines recommend a value of 330 ms or less.[21] Given the limited information available on the mechanism of action and the incidence and relevance of reduced drug-induced AP duration, the proarrhythmic threshold for acquired SQTS has yet to be truly established. Other ECG findings for SQTS can include absent ST-segments and tall, narrow, symmetrical T waves.[17] Clinical suspicion for congenital SQTS is often heightened after unexplained syncope in an otherwise healthy individual, episodes of atrial fibrillation, polymorphic ventricular tachycardia, ventricular fibrillation, or a family history of unexplained sudden cardiac death.[17]

Treatment

Because of the rarity of SQTS, not much is known about successful treatment. Similar to LQTS, if drug-induced SQTS is suspected, removal of the noxious drug is prudent.

Some reports have indicated that quinidine administration has been effective in increasing repolarization time in those with the congenital form of SQTS[22,23]; however, drug therapy options, specifically directed at prolonging cardiac repolarization, require further study. Primary and secondary therapy for confirmed symptomatic congenital SQTS subjects is implantable cardioverter-defibrillator (ICD) (class 1 recommendation).[17]

ANTIARRHYTHMICS AND PROARRHYTHMIA

Antiarrhythmics are a class of drugs used to treat arrhythmias; however, they also have the potential to cause arrhythmias, also known as a proarrhythmics. Proposed by Singh and Vaughan Williams,[24] antiarrhythmics are typically divided into drug groups based on their mechanisms of action (**Table 2**). The effects of class III drugs and their mechanisms of action on potassium ion channels have been shown in the discussion with acquired LQTS.

Class I, Sodium Channel Blockade Arrhythmias

The unintended adverse effects of cardiac drugs, especially sodium channel blockers (NCBs), have most prominently been shown in the early 1990s with the results of the Cardiac Arrhythmia Suppression Trial (CAST).[25,26] The CAST was a seminal study that tested whether suppression of premature ventricular complexes with NCBs reduced mortality in subjects experiencing myocardial infarction. Unexpectedly, investigators found that the rate of mortality was higher in subjects randomized to receive the study drug. Of the 183 deaths recorded within the study, 66% (n = 122) were determined to be due to arrhythmia.[27] Although the exact electrophysiologic mechanism underlying these deaths is unknown, it is thought that the administration of NCBs slows conduction through established ischemic zones of tissue, thereby facilitating pathways for re-entrant ventricular arrhythmias.

Class 1 antiarrhythmic drugs work by inhibiting the action of the voltage-gated sodium channel, active during phase 0 of the myocardial AP. Pacemaker cells (SA and AV nodal cells) do not rely on sodium channels for depolarization and are therefore unaffected by administration of NCBs. In myocardial cells, blocking sodium channels causes the rate and rise of depolarization currents to be decreased, reducing the potential conduction velocity throughout the myocardium—an important element in

Table 2
Classification of antiarrhythmics

Class	Action	Drug Examples
I	Acts on the sodium channel Subtypes: 1a, 1b, 1c	Quinidine, procainamide, phenytoin, lidocaine, flecainide, moricizine, disopyramide
II	Antisympathetic agent (BB)	Carvedilol, propranolol, metoprolol, atenolol, esmolol
III	Alters potassium channel action	Amiodarone,[a] sotalol,[b] dofetilide, dronedarone, ibutilide
IV	Alters calcium channel action	Verapamil, diltiazem
V	Other/unknown mechanism of action	Adenosine, digoxin, magnesium sulfate

[a] Amiodarone has class I-IV activity.
[b] Sotalol has class II activity.
Data from Singh BN, Vaughan Williams EM. The effect of amiodarone, a new anti-anginal drug, on cardiac muscle. Br J Pharmacol 1970;39(4):657–67.

suppressing re-entry arrhythmias. Currently, there are 3 classes of NCBs (1a, 1b, 1c), each with different effects on the different phases of repolarization within the AP. Similar to LQTS, although not an acquired arrhythmia, Brugada syndrome is a congenital disorder that affects the sodium ion channel. With this genetic mutation, the influx of sodium during phase 0 of the AP is reduced, altering cardiac depolarization. Subsequently, this alters cardiac repolarization, causing increased heterogeneity across the myocardium and provides the substrate necessary for re-entry arrhythmias.[28] Brugada syndrome is characterized by a coved-type elevated ST-segment in the right precordial leads (V_1 to V_3) and is associated with an increased risk for sudden death.[29] Importantly, because administration of NCBs exaggerates the effect of sodium ion dysfunction, in patients with Brugada syndrome, close electrocardiograph monitoring is needed.

Clinical features

A slowing of the upslope of depolarization within the AP results in widening of the QRS complex on an ECG. Other electrocardiographic findings may be a right bundle branch pattern, R-wave elevation in lead aVR, and right-axis deviation.[30] Toxicity may also cause slowing of the intraventricular conduction, creating the substrate for unidirectional conduction block and possibly a re-entry circuit. In this state, ventricular tachycardia can develop and degenerate into ventricular fibrillation and asystole.[31]

Treatment

NCB toxicity can be exhibited by any drug that has sodium channel blocking effects, that is, tricyclic antidepressants, cocaine, or quinidine. Similar to other drug-induced arrhythmias, treatment initially centers on removing the noxious drug. To prevent tachyarrhythmias from developing, studies have shown a beneficial effect with increasing the serum pH through administration of sodium bicarbonate.[32–35] Importantly, if cardioversion is used for the treatment of ventricular tachycardia, NCBs may increase resistance, resulting in recurrence arrhythmia soon after. In patients with Brugada syndrome, treatment options are limited to the placement of an ICD; however, as with cardioversion, these devices present their own unique challenges related to the administration of NCBs. In patients with ICDs or external cardioverter-defibrillators, NCBs, such as lidocaine and mexiletine, increase the energy required for successful defibrillation. This is known as the defibrillation threshold and is defined as the lowest energy needed to restore sinus activity.[36] Increasing defibrillation threshold impairs a defibrillator's ability to successfully terminate a ventricular tachyarrhythmia. It is thought that a decrease in sodium channel function increases the stimulus strength required to initiate an AP. One proposed mechanism for arrhythmia is that NCBs and defibrillation both slow conduction velocity and alter the refractory period. Heterogeneity in conduction and refractoriness results, producing the substrate for re-entrant arrhythmias immediately after a shock, resulting in failed defibrillation.

Class IV, Calcium Channel Blockade Arrhythmias

Pacemaker cells, unlike myocardial cells, depolarize because of slow inward calcium currents. Calcium channel blockers (CCBs) act by inhibiting the flow of extracellular calcium into the cell. When this occurs, contractility is reduced, and SA node and AV node conduction are slowed. Although all CCBs act on calcium ion channels, each subclass acts on different aspects of the ion channel, resulting in functional differences, particularly with regard to their vasodilator potency and inotropic, chronotropic, and dromotropic effects.[37] There are 2 main subclasses of

CCBs: dihydropyridines (DHP) and nondihydropyridines (non-DHP) (**Table 3**). One of the major adverse arrhythmic effects of CCBs, especially with administration of DHPs, is reflex tachycardia. With a reduction in arterial blood pressure due to smooth muscle dilation, baroreceptors within the aortic arch signal the medulla oblongata to increase sympathetic stimulation. This increase in sympathetic stimulation results in a rapid increase in heart rate and stroke volume. For patients with myocardial ischemia, this is especially problematic because the increased oxygen demand can extend ischemic events. Another condition that warrants hypervigilance when administering a CCB is SA node dysfunction. Patients with SA node dysfunction are sensitive to CCBs effects, especially with verapamil, because of the inhibitory activity; this can lead to severe arrhythmias, such as sinus bradycardia and SA node arrest.[38] A congenital cause of severe arrhythmia with CCB administration is in the presence of pre-excitation syndrome, known commonly as WPW.[7] In the normal heart, impulse conduction from the atria is spread to the ventricles through the AV node-His-Purkinje system. The AV node acts protectively to slow conduction, preventing one-to-one conduction from the atria to the ventricles, and is especially important in the presence of atrial tachyarrhythmias. In WPW syndrome, abnormal conductive cardiac tissue bridges the atria and the ventricles, providing a rapid pathway that preempts AV node conduction, allowing for one-to-one conduction outside the normal pathway.[39] Therefore, with administration of CCBs, AV nodal conduction is slowed, facilitating antegrade conduction over the accessory pathway. For this reason, use of non-DHP CCBs in a patient with atrial fibrillation and pre-excitation can potentially be life-threatening and is therefore contraindicated.

Clinical features

Clinical features of CCB toxicity are closely related to their course of action on the AP of pacemaker and myocardial cells. As calcium influx is attenuated, bradycardia, SA node arrest, or first-, second-, or third-degree blocks can develop. Bundle branch blocks may also be present on the ECG.

Treatment

Toxicity with CCBs requires supportive care based on symptoms and drug-activity duration (because of sustained-release formulations). Vasopressive agents and intravenous fluids may be indicated to counter hypotension as well as atropine to improve contractility and heart rate. For further treatment options the reader is referred to the comprehensive review by Graudins and colleagues.[40]

Table 3
Calcium channel blocker classifications

Drug Group	Action	Drug Examples
DHP	Reduces systemic vascular resistance and arterial pressure	Amlodipine, nifedipine, felodipine, nicardipine
Non-DHP		
Phenylalkylamines	Selective for myocardium: reduces oxygen demand, negative inotropy	Verapamil, gallopamil, fendiline
Benzothiazepines	Intermediate: some DHP and phenylalkylamine activity	Diltiazem
Nonselective	Varied mechanisms of action	Bepridil, mibefradil, gabapentin

Class V, Other and Unknown Mechanisms of Action

Adenosine is a naturally occurring, rapidly metabolized compound that produces bradycardia due to AV nodal conduction delay and a negative chronotropic action on the sinus node. It is widely used as an antiarrhythmic agent for the acute management of re-entrant supraventricular tachycardia (SVT) involving the AV node.[41] It has also been used to differentiate between wide QRS complex SVT versus ventricular tachycardia and to unmask the presence of concealed bypass tracts. Atrial fibrillation is the most common persistent proarrhythmic effect of adenosine[42] and is caused by atrial-AP shortening and reduced atrial refractoriness.[42] Other expected side effects of administration of adenosine are long pauses and bradyarrhythmias. In the AV node, adenosine prolongs AV nodal refractoriness and suppresses nodal excitability, resulting in AV conduction block[43]; this may progress to sinus arrest and complete heart block in cases with pre-existing sinus node dysfunction or conduction abnormality. Besides bradyarrhythmias, reflex tachyarrhythmias may also develop after adenosine administration.[44,45] The pathophysiologic mechanism of ventricular ectopy is thought to be secondary to increased circulating catecholamine levels and an increase in sympathetic tone. Because of adenosine's very short half-life (<10 seconds), after-administration electrophysiologic changes are most commonly transient; however, in the presence of symptomatic bradyarrhythmias, transcutaneous pacing may be warranted.

Class II, Antisympathetic Agents

β-Blockers (BBs) are a class II antiarrhythmic and work by blocking myocardial β-adrenoceptors.[40] These receptors contribute to a cascade of cellular actions that open a specific ion channel called L-type calcium ion channels. Administration of a BB reduces calcium influx into the myocardial cell, reducing the strength and speed of contractility. A small subset of BBs (propranolol and labetalol) also has an inhibitory action on sodium ion channels, displaying to a lesser degree some class I activity.[40] The major arrhythmia related to BBs is bradycardia. Toxicity with BBs with class I activity may also demonstrate a widening of the QRS complex on an ECG, due to inhibition of depolarizing currents. Similar to CCBs, treatment of BBs' toxicity is aimed at countering subsequent bradycardia and reduced contractility.

SUMMARY

Cardiac function is dependent on normal electrical and mechanical activity. Pacemaker and myocardial cells provide the stimulus and the contractile units that are responsible for these functions. Many drugs administered to alleviate disease also have the negative side effect of altering cardiac function. At the cellular level, these drugs often block or interact with ion channel functioning and most commonly impact cardiac repolarization. Understanding the different cell compositions and functions within the heart allow for an understanding of their different APs. This is important to understanding how drugs can interact and cause arrhythmias. Drug-induced arrhythmias are an important, adverse effect of drug treatment. The underlying mechanisms responsible for the proarrhythmic effects of various cardiovascular and noncardiovascular drugs are complex. Understanding cardiac electrophysiology, mechanisms of drug actions, and contributory factors like electrolyte imbalance and disease is critical to understanding the development of arrhythmias and their effective treatment strategies.

ACKNOWLEDGMENTS

The authors thank Peter Van Dam and Eric Helfenbein for the development and use of illustrations, as well as Angela Tsiperfal for kindly reviewing the article.

REFERENCES

1. Frommeyer G, Eckardt L. Drug-induced proarrhythmia: risk factors and electrophysiological mechanisms. Nat Rev Cardiol 2016;13(1):36–47.
2. Selzer A, Wray HW. Quinidine syncope: paroxysmal ventricular fibrillation occurring during treatment of chronic atrial arrhythmias. Circulation 1964;30(1):17–26.
3. Dash D. Proarrhythmia (secondary). In: Kibos A, Knight B, Essebag V, et al, editors. Cardiac arrhythmias. Verlag (London): Springer; 2014. p. 345–50.
4. Heist EK, Ruskin JN. Drug-induced arrhythmia. Circulation 2010;122(14):1426–35.
5. Ottoboni LK, Lee A, Zei P. Cardiac anatomy, physiology, electrophysiology, and pharmacology. Cardiac arrhythmia management. Ames (Iowa): John Wiley & Sons, Ltd.; 2011. p. 1–24.
6. Mani BC, Pavri BB. Dual atrioventricular nodal pathways physiology: a review of relevant anatomy, electrophysiology, and electrocardiographic manifestations. Indian Pacing Electrophysiol J 2014;14(1):12–25.
7. Wolff L, Parkinson J, White PD. Bundle-branch block with short P-R interval in healthy young people prone to paroxysmal tachycardia. Am Heart J 1930;5(6):685–704.
8. van Noord C, Eijgelsheim M, Stricker BH. Drug- and non-drug-associated QT interval prolongation. Br J Clin Pharmacol 2010;70(1):16–23.
9. Pickham D, Helfenbein E, Shinn JA, et al. High prevalence of corrected QT interval prolongation in acutely ill patients is associated with mortality: results of the QT in Practice (QTIP) Study. Crit Care Med 2012;40(2):394–9.
10. Pickham D, Helfenbein E, Shinn JA, et al. How many patients need QT interval monitoring in critical care units? Preliminary report of the QT in Practice Study. J Electrocardiol 2010;43(6):572–6.
11. Drew BJ, Ackerman MJ, Funk M, et al. Prevention of torsade de pointes in hospital settings: a scientific statement from the American Heart Association and the American College of Cardiology Foundation endorsed by the American Association of Critical-Care Nurses and the International Society for Computerized Electrocardiology. J Am Coll Cardiol 2010;55(9):934–47.
12. Roden DM. Acquired long QT syndromes and the risk of proarrhythmia. J Cardiovasc Electrophysiol 2000;11(8):938–40.
13. Kannankeril PJ, Roden DM, Norris KJ, et al. Genetic susceptibility to acquired long QT syndrome: pharmacologic challenge in first-degree relatives. Heart Rhythm 2010;2(2):134–40.
14. Fazekas T, Scherlag BJ, Vos M, et al. Magnesium and the heart: antiarrhythmic therapy with magnesium. Clin Cardiol 1993;16(11):768–74.
15. Viskin S. Torsades de pointes. Curr Treat Options Cardiovasc Med 1999;1(2):187–95.
16. Gussak I, Brugada P, Brugada J, et al. Idiopathic short QT interval: a new clinical syndrome? Cardiology 2000;94(2):99–102.
17. Anzelevitch C, Cordeiro J. Short QT syndrome. In: Link M, editor. UpToDate; 2015.
18. Goldberger AL. Cardiac arrhythmias due to digoxin toxicity. In: Traub S, editor. UpToDate; 2015.

19. Smith TW. Digitalis. Mechanisms of action and clinical use. N Engl J Med 1988; 318(6):358–65.
20. Malik M. Facts, fancies and follies of drug-induced QT/QTc interval shortening. Br J Pharmacol 2010;159(1):70–6.
21. Priori SG, Wilde AA, Horie M, et al. HRS/EHRA/APHRS expert consensus statement on the diagnosis and management of patients with inherited primary arrhythmia syndromes: document endorsed by HRS, EHRA, and APHRS in May 2013 and by ACCF, AHA, PACES, and AEPC in June 2013. Heart Rhythm 2013;10(12):1932–63.
22. Giustetto C, Schimpf R, Mazzanti A, et al. Long-term follow-up of patients with short QT syndrome. J Am Coll Cardiol 2011;58(6):587–95.
23. Kaufman ES. Quinidine in short QT syndrome: an old drug for a new disease. J Cardiovasc Electrophysiol 2007;18(6):665–6.
24. Singh BN, Vaughan Williams EM. The effect of amiodarone, a new anti-anginal drug, on cardiac muscle. Br J Pharmacol 1970;39(4):657–67.
25. Preliminary report: effect of encainide and flecainide on mortality in a randomized trial of arrhythmia suppression after myocardial infarction. N Engl J Med 1989; 321(6):406–12.
26. Effect of the antiarrhythmic agent moricizine on survival after myocardial infarction. N Engl J Med 1992;327(4):227–33.
27. Epstein AE, Bigger JT Jr, Wyse DG, et al. Events in the Cardiac Arrhythmia Suppression Trial (CAST): mortality in the entire population enrolled. J Am Coll Cardiol 1991;18(1):14–9.
28. Weiss R, Barmada MM, Nguyen T, et al. Clinical and molecular heterogeneity in the Brugada syndrome: a novel gene locus on chromosome 3. Circulation 2002; 105(6):707–13.
29. Brugada P, Brugada J. Right bundle branch block, persistent ST segment elevation and sudden cardiac death: a distinct clinical and electrocardiographic syndrome. A multicenter report. J Am Coll Cardiol 1992;20(6):1391–6.
30. Lionte C, Bologa C, Sorodoc L. Toxic and drug-induced changes of the electrocardiogram. In: Millis RM, editor. Advances in electrocardiograms—clinical applications. InTech; 2012. p. 271–97. Available at: http://www.intech.com/.
31. Brugada J, Boersma L, Kirchhof C, et al. Proarrhythmic effects of flecainide. Experimental evidence for increased susceptibility to reentrant arrhythmias. Circulation 1991;84(4):1808–18.
32. Di Grande A, Giuffrida C, Narbone G, et al. Management of sodium-channel blocker poisoning: the role of hypertonic sodium salts. Eur Rev Med Pharmacol Sci 2010;14(1):25–30.
33. Courand PY, Sibellas F, Ranc S, et al. Arrhythmogenic effect of flecainide toxicity. Cardiol J 2013;20(2):203–5.
34. Chouty F, Funck-Brentano C, Landau JM, et al. Efficacy of high doses of molar lactate by the venous route in flecainide poisoning. Presse Med 1987;16(17): 808–10 [in French].
35. Bajaj AK, Woosley RL, Roden DM. Acute electrophysiologic effects of sodium administration in dogs treated with O-desmethyl encainide. Circulation 1989; 80(4):994–1002.
36. Dopp AL, Miller JM, Tisdale JE. Effect of drugs on defibrillation capacity. Drugs 2008;68(5):607–30.
37. Abernethy DR, Schwartz JB. Calcium-antagonist drugs. N Engl J Med 1999; 341(19):1447–57.

38. Ramoska EA, Spiller HA, Myers A. Calcium channel blocker toxicity. Ann Emerg Med 1990;19(6):649–53.
39. Lauer M, Sung R. Anatomy and physiology of the conduction system. In: Podrid P, Kowey P, editors. Cardiac arrhythmia: mechanisms, diagnosis, and management. 2nd edition. New York: Lippincott; 2001. p. 17–8.
40. Graudins A, Lee HM, Druda D. Calcium channel antagonist and beta-blocker overdose: antidotes and adjunct therapies. Br J Clin Pharmacol 2015;81(3): 453–61.
41. Mallet ML. Proarrhythmic effects of adenosine: a review of the literature. Emerg Med J 2004;21(4):408–10.
42. Kabell G, Buchanan LV, Gibson JK, et al. Effects of adenosine on atrial refractoriness and arrhythmias. Cardiovasc Res 1994;28(9):1385–9.
43. Russo V, Nigro G, Papa AA, et al. Adenosine-induced sinus tachycardia in a patient with myotonic dystrophy type 1. Acta Myol 2014;33(2):104–6.
44. Tan HL, Spekhorst HH, Peters RJ, et al. Adenosine induced ventricular arrhythmias in the emergency room. Pacing Clin Electrophysiol 2001;24(4 Pt 1):450–5.
45. Misra D, Van Tosh A, Schweitzer P. Adenosine induced monomorphic ventricular tachycardia. Pacing Clin Electrophysiol 2000;23(6):1044–6.

Arrhythmias and Cardiac Bedside Monitoring in the Neonatal Intensive Care Unit

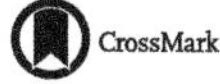

Sherri L. McMullen, PhD, FNP, NNP-BC[a,b,*]

KEYWORDS

- Cardiac monitoring • Neonatal intensive care unit • Electrocardiography • Infants • Neonates

KEY POINTS

- It is essential to comprehend the cardiovascular changes that occur in an infant after birth and to understand important information provided on a neonate's bedside monitor.
- Caregivers must understand the physiology surrounding arrhythmias and the importance of reporting a variance from baseline.
- A specialized bedside monitor can offer early warning signs of late-onset sepsis using an algorithm and the subtle changes in heart rate and rhythm.

INTRODUCTION

In 1963, Patrick Bouvier Kennedy, son of President John F. Kennedy, died as a result of complications from being born 5 weeks early.[1] Today, 50 years later, he would have a greater than 95% chance of survival. Neonatal care impacts our country greatly because one in every 10 infants is born preterm in the United States.[2] Despite this remarkable improvement in patient outcomes, in 2010, the infant mortality rates in the United States remain 3 times higher than that of countries with the lowest mortalities (6.05 per 1000 live births).[3] The care provided to critically ill infants over the last 50 years has dramatically improved survival as a result of the advancements in knowledge and technology; however, we must continue our efforts to reduce infant mortality. One way to further reduce it is to improve our knowledge and surveillance of infants in the neonatal intensive care unit (NICU). Cardiac monitors provide information about respiration, heart rate variability, and arrhythmias; in addition, with the use of specialized bedside monitors, early signs of sepsis can be recognized. The purpose of this article is to review neonatal cardiac physiology, to examine neonatal arrhythmias

The author has nothing to disclose.
[a] College of Nursing, Upstate Medical University, 750 East Adams Street, Syracuse, NY 13210, USA; [b] Nursing Practice, University of Rochester Medical Center, 150 Crittenden Boulevard, Rochester, NY 14642, USA
* Upstate Medical University, 750 East Adams Street, Syracuse, NY 13210.
E-mail address: McMulleS@Upstate.edu

Crit Care Nurs Clin N Am 28 (2016) 373–386
http://dx.doi.org/10.1016/j.cnc.2016.04.008 ccnursing.theclinics.com
0899-5885/16/$ – see front matter © 2016 Elsevier Inc. All rights reserved.

visible on the bedside monitor, and to describe a specialized bedside monitor that provides data indicating early signs of sepsis.

THE PHYSIOLOGY OF A NEONATE: THE FIRST 28 DAYS OF LIFE

A neonate is a human newborn in the first 28 days of life. It is important to understand the transition from fetal to newborn circulation when performing a cardiac evaluation. Fetal circulation has high pulmonary pressures, which divert blood from the pulmonary beds and into the patent ductus arteriosus. Although not evident on the bedside monitor, high pulmonary pressure leads to right ventricular (RV) dominance and should be a consideration when interpreting the newborn electrocardiogram (ECG). This RV dominance is not always evident in preterm infants depending on their birth gestational ages: the closer to 40 weeks the infant is born, the more evident the RV dominance.[4] What is evident on the bedside monitors is the heart rate and a variance in heart rate, and that variance should be noted by the nurse. The median heart rate for newborn infants is 127 beats per minute (bpm); the rate increases over the first month of age to 145 bpm before decreasing over the next few years.[5] This rate can be lower when sleeping and higher with crying. Institutions have individual guidelines for low and high limits for neonatal bedside cardiac monitoring, which are based on the diagnoses an infant has on admission to the NICU. These limits can vary; for example, in a level II NICU, a limit of 80 bpm and 200 bpm may be acceptable if the unit does not have a large number of very premature infants (born before 27 weeks' gestation) and high acuity. Whereas, a level III NICU, with a large number of very premature infants with very low birth weight (fewer than 1500 g), may desire a level of 100 bpm and 250 bpm.

In the normal electrical conduction system, the impulse, which originates in the sinoatrial (SA) node located within the right atrium, activates the right and the left atrium, and the atria contract simultaneously. The atria contract and blood flows into the ventricles; the impulse continues to the atrioventricular (AV) node where it is delayed, which allows for filling of the ventricles. The impulse continues through the bundle of His, the bundle branches, and spontaneously terminates among the Purkinje fibers leading to an organized, simultaneous contraction of both ventricles. After the cardiac muscle contracts (depolarizes), there is a period of rest wherein the tissue cannot be excited to contract again (repolarization).

THE NORMAL ELECTROCARDIOGRAM OF THE NEONATE HEART

The neonatal sinus rhythm ECG has a P wave (atrial depolarization) before every QRS (ventricular depolarization), and this is followed by a T wave (ventricular repolarization). The QRS duration is shorter in infants than adults as a result of the reduced cardiac muscle mass.[6] The PR interval displays AV conduction and is the measurement from the onset of the P wave to the onset of the QRS complex (ventricular depolarization). The QT interval begins at the onset of the QRS and ends at the end of the T wave. The QT interval duration changes with heart rate, is age dependent, and is represented by the QT_c identifying the correction for heart rate.[7] The R-R interval is measured from the beginning of one QRS complex to the beginning of the next QRS complex. Many of these intervals are difficult to appreciate on a neonatal bedside monitor, especially with tachyarrhythmias because the heart rates are much faster than children and adults, which make the intervals much smaller.

The electrical axis is the direction the electrical impulse flows. Although there is a T and P wave axis, the QRS complex is the most important axis to determine. In a neonate with normal sinus rhythm, atrial depolarization occurs from the SA node and the impulse flows right to left and top to bottom. The QRS complex is predominantly upright or positive in both limb leads I and aVF, and then the QRS complex axis is normal. A task force of the European Society of Cardiology reports that an axis deviation is seen in a variety of abnormalities, including AV septal defect, ventricular septal defect, tricuspid atresia, and Wolff-Parkinson-White (WPW) syndrome (a condition with an extra electrical pathway) but may be occasionally observed in otherwise normal neonates.[8]

Electrocardiogram Leads

The bedside cardiac monitor is a monitoring tool used by caregivers in the NICU to monitor critically ill neonates (**Fig. 1**). Lead placement is an important factor in interpreting the bedside monitor ECG. The placement of the 3 electrodes with the bedside monitor can vary among clinicians, and placement will change the pattern of the ECG. The monitor's manufacturing recommendations should be followed closely; the electrodes must not touch each other to obtain proper data. Electrodes can be placed on the chest or limb leads can be used if there is a dermatologic problem or, with extremely premature infants, to reduce skin breakdown. Electrodes should not be placed over the nipples or over broken or bruised skin. Caution should be exercised when removing electrodes to reduce skin damage. Of note, recent efforts have focused on the development of unobtrusive ECG monitoring by embedding electrodes into the mattress of the premature infant. This technology uses capacitive sensing array technology to obtain ECG information for care providers without the need for electrodes being placed directly on the skin of the infant.[9]

CARDIAC ARRHYTHMIAS IN THE NEONATE HEART

It is important for the bedside NICU nurse to be aware of the information a cardiac monitor offers and of the responsibility to report any variance from baseline. Special

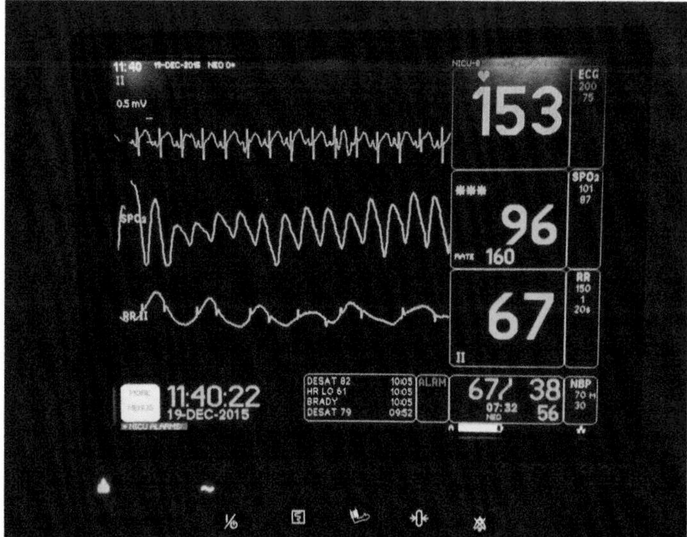

Fig. 1. A NICU bedside monitor. The top display and number is the ECG; the second display and number is the oxygen saturation; the third display and number is the respiratory rate; the bottom number without a display is the last recorded blood pressure.

attention and observation should be given to those infants who have a history of an arrhythmia while in utero. Those fetuses who were treated for a fetal arrhythmia in utero may have a recurrence in fetal arrhythmia when the level of a medication decreases after delivery.[7] The incidence of arrhythmias in neonates ranges from 1% to 5%.[10] More recently, a retrospective database search of 662,698 live births over 20 years documented an incidence of 24.4 per 100,000 live births (0.02%).[11] Badrawi and colleagues[12] reported the incidence of arrhythmia in the NICU as 8.5% for benign and 1.5% for nonbenign arrhythmias. The distribution of arrhythmias was as follows: supraventricular tachycardia (SVT) (n = 3), ventricular tachycardia (n = 1), second-degree AV heart block (n = 1), complete AV heart block (n = 1), and arrhythmia secondary to hyperkalemia (n = 1) (**Fig. 2**).[12] Arrhythmias can be associated with congenital heart disease, and a normal 12-lead ECG cannot rule out congenital heart disease.[7] The neonatal ECG varies from the adult ECG; adult standards cannot be used when interpreting an infant ECG. There is great variability after birth, and it is important to understand normal values when interpreting the neonatal ECG. If there is concern about the heart rate or rhythm on the bedside monitor, a resting standard 12-lead ECG should be obtained and interpreted by an experienced practitioner. Normal ECG values depend on age, and it is outside the scope of the bedside NICU nurse to know these normal values for the first year of life.[13] The clinical impact of an arrhythmia on an infant depends on the baseline clinical status of the infant and the type of arrhythmia present.

CLASSIFICATION OF ARRHYTHMIAS

An arrhythmia is an abnormal rhythm, and there is no uniformity of classification for neonatal arrhythmias. Some classify arrhythmias according to rhythm, such as tachyarrhythmias or bradyarrhythmias (**Table 1**).[12,14] A benign arrhythmia is considered non–life threatening and without the need for immediate intervention or without evidence of future health problems, whereas a nonbenign arrhythmia is sudden and requires immediate recognition and treatment for optimal patient outcomes.[12]

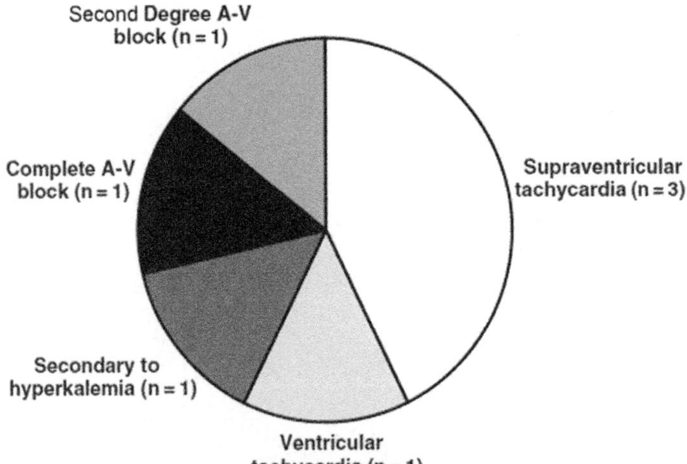

Fig. 2. Frequency distribution of arrhythmias. (*From* Badrawi N, Hegazy R, Tikovic E, et al. Arrhythmia in the neonatal intensive care unit. Pediatric Cardiology 2009;30:328; with permission.)

Table 1
Classification of cardiac rhythms

Benign Rhythms	Nonbenign Rhythms
Bradycardia	Supraventricular tachycardia
Tachycardia	WPW
Premature atrial contractions	Atrial flutter
Premature ventricular contractions	Heart block
Nodal or junctional rhythm	Ventricular tachycardia
	Ventricular fibrillation
	Long QT syndrome
	Sudden infant death syndrome

Benign Arrhythmias

Sinus bradycardia

One common type of bradyarrhythmia is sinus bradycardia, and this is commonly seen on the bedside monitor in the NICU. Sinus bradycardia is defined as a heartbeat 2 standard deviations less than the mean or fewer than 80 bpm.[14] Transient sinus bradycardia in a premature infant can be a result of an episode of apnea (cessation of breathing for 20 seconds or longer) and an immature central nervous system.[15] Many additional causes of bradycardia exist, including hypoxemia and acidosis; hypoxia causes sinus bradycardia by depolarizing the membrane potential. **Box 1** contains a further listing of causes of neonatal sinus bradycardia. Infants with bradycardia should be evaluated to rule out a diagnosis of long QT syndrome (LQTS).[14]

Sinus tachycardia

Neonatal sinus tachycardia is a sinus rhythm that is greater than the upper limit of normal and increases during the first month (166–179).[7] Tachycardia can be a result of irritability and crying or fever, sepsis, dehydration, pain, and anemia.[7] Other causes

Box 1
Causes of neonatal sinus bradycardia

- Apnea
- Central nervous abnormalities
- Hypothermia
- Hypopituitarism
- Increased intracranial pressure
- Increase in vagal tone, including pharyngeal stimulation
- Gastric distention
- Upper airway obstruction
- Medications
- Valsalva maneuver
- Oversedation
- Hypothyroidism

Data from Refs.[7,8,14]

of sinus tachycardia can include hyperthyroidism or the use of medications, such as bronchodilators or beta-adrenergic agonists.

Premature atrial contractions

Premature atrial contractions (PACs) are the most common arrhythmias found during the neonatal time and are characterized by a premature electrical impulse originating within the atria.[16] The ECG shows an early sinus beat preceded by a normal or inverted P wave and a pause following the premature beat. Sometimes, if the interval between beats is shortened, the electrical activity is not transmitted because the refractory period of the ventricles and QRS complex does not follow a PAC. The QRS is narrow because the conduction follows the normal conduction system. A central venous line advanced into the right atrium can cause PACs, and the line should be repositioned to the correct position. Usually, PACs resolve within a few days. If they do not resolve spontaneously within a few weeks, follow-up should be arranged with a pediatric cardiologist.[8,17]

Premature ventricular contractions

Premature ventricular contractions (PVCs) are premature electrical impulses from the ventricles, which lead to an early and, in most cases, extra beat. Because they do not originate in the SA node, PVCs are not preceded by a P wave and have a widened QRS because the impulse travels outside the normal ventricular conduction system. There is usually a compensatory pause after the PVC. The extra electrical impulse causes the SA node to be refractory to the next regular beat. When a PVC is present with every other beat, the pattern is labeled ventricular bigeminy; if a PVC is present with every third beat, the pattern is labeled ventricular trigeminy. Most infants with PVCs have structurally normal hearts, and no pharmacologic treatment is usually necessary.[10] Frequent PVCs can be an indication of an underlying cardiac problem.

Nodal or junctional rhythm

A nodal rhythm originates within the bundle of His, and a junctional rhythm originates within the AV node. The AV node can become the primary pacemaker of the heart at a much slower pace if the SA node fails to control the rhythm. Because the rhythm does not originate within the ventricles, the QRS complex is narrow.

Nonbenign Arrhythmias

Supraventricular tachycardia

SVT is one of the most common arrhythmias in infants and has an incidence of 1:250 (**Fig. 3**).[12,18,19] The heart rate can be between 220 and 280 bpm.[20] Accessory AV conduction or AV node reentrant tachycardia is the most common causes of SVT.[18,21] A reentrant rhythm involves 2 pathways, one unidirectional impulse and one impulse that is blocked, so the impulse reenters from another direction (retrograde).[21] If the tissue is in the refractory period, the impulse will die; however, if the tissue is excitable, the impulse is conducted and can lead to contraction of the tissue.

Wolff-Parkinson-White

WPW is a form of tachycardia resulting from an accessory pathway (**Fig. 4**).[18,21] Global reentry is the reentry model on a larger scale, such as between the atria and ventricles. Instead of the impulse traveling from the AV node to the ventricles, accessory pathways exist from the SA node sending additional impulses.[21] There can also be local AV nodal reentry, which provides an impulse back to the AV node; this rate can stimulate the ventricle and lead to SVT.[21] The incidence has been reported to be between 0.4 and 1.0 per 1000 in infants and children, with 60% being diagnosed within the first

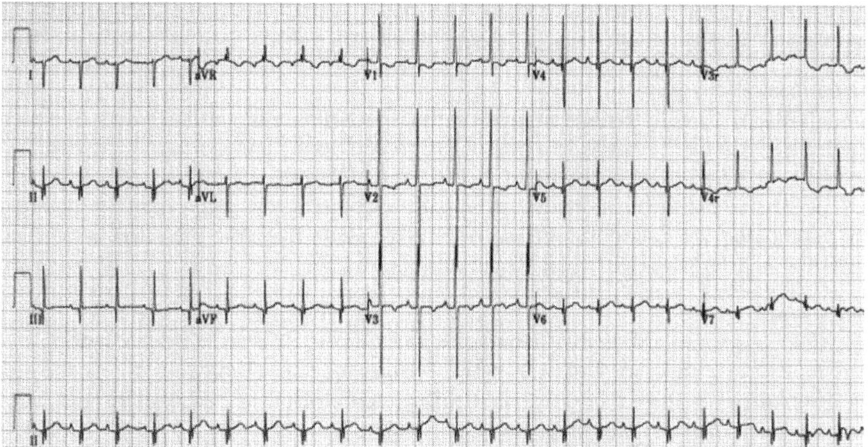

Fig. 3. A normal 12-lead ECG of a 1-week-old infant. (*From* Resuscitation education. How to read the paediatric ECG. 2011. Available at: http://www.resus.com.au/ecg-gallery/. Accessed February 11, 2016; with permission.)

2 months of age.[22] Three characteristic ECG findings of WPW include a shortened PR interval, the presence of a delta wave, and a widened QRS complex.[20] The electrical impulse travels through both the AV node and an accessory pathway, known as the bundle of Kent.[20] These two impulses lead to ventricular preexcitation causing depolarization and tachycardia. SVT is the most common arrhythmia associated with WPW,

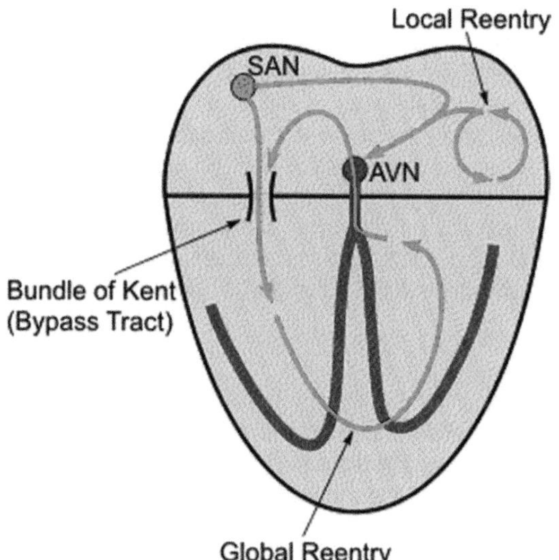

Fig. 4. Physiology of WPW, global and local reentry impulse pathways. The normal impulse travels from the AV node (AVN) to the ventricles (*red lines*). When an accessory impulse originates from the SA node (SAN), additional impulses exist (*green lines*), creating additional impulses at a much faster rate than normally present without these accessory ones. (*From* Klabunde R. Cardiovascular physiology concepts. 2013. Available at: www.cvphysiology.com/Arrhythmias/A008c.htm. Accessed January 15, 2016; with permission.)

so WPW should be ruled out in all cases presenting with SVT because untreated WPW can lead to sudden death from ventricular fibrillation.[20,23]

Atrial flutter

Atrial flutter is considered an uncommon rhythm of a neonate and is evidenced by a sawtooth pattern of P waves at a rate of 240 to 360 bpm.[7] The incidence has been reported as 2.1 per 100,000 live births.[11] The ventricular rate is variable and can be 1:1, 2:1, or 3:1 and depends on the atrial beats conducted across the AV node. Reducing the ventricular rate is important to allow time for ventricular filling to improve cardiac output. It is considered an atrial reentrant abnormality.

Heart block

Heart block is a rare arrhythmia; in one prospective study, it was found that among 457 infants, 2 (0.4%) had a form of heart block.[12] Heart block is a bradyarrhythmia and can be identified on a bedside monitor. Like adult heart block, it is classified as first-, second-, or third-degree heart block and can be either congenital or acquired.[7] Congenital complete AV block is associated with a maternal systematic lupus erythematosus or Sjögren syndrome diagnosis. The anti-Ro (Sjögren syndrome, SS-A) and anti-La (Sjögren syndrome, SS-B) antibodies associated with lupus are transmitted across the placenta to the fetus and thought to disrupt the conduction system during fetal development.[7]

- First-degree heart block is identified by a prolonged PR interval on the ECG. This prolonged interval is a result of the delay in conduction between the atria and ventricles.
- Second-degree heart block is an intermittent conduction failure and is divided into 2 categories: type I (Wenckebach) and type II (Mobitz).[7] In type I, the conduction progressively slows until the impulse ceases with a lengthened PR interval and then a dropped QRS complex; in type II, there is an abrupt failure of atrial conduction without a prolonged PR interval, which can progress into complete heart block, a life-threatening condition.
- In third-degree or complete heart block or AV dissociation, there is no conduction between the atrium and ventricles with a random PR interval.
- Less severe forms of heart block can be asymptomatic; in more severe forms, congestive heart failure can develop or death can result. When a low heart rate is audible (<60 bpm), assessment of the infant is most important. This point is especially true in the rare case of heart block in the delivery room to avoid interventions, such as cardiopulmonary resuscitation, if not necessary.

Ventricular tachycardia

Ventricular tachycardia is rare in the neonate and has been reported as 0.8 per 100,000 live births.[11] It can be difficult to differentiate SVT from ventricular tachycardia on a bedside cardiac monitor unless looking very closely at the monitor. Although the QRS complex is narrow in SVT, it is widened in ventricular tachycardia; however, when ventricular tachycardia is present, it is considered a medical emergency because it can progress into ventricular fibrillation and death.

Ventricular fibrillation

Ventricular fibrillation is a dysfunction and incoordination of the ventricles, which leads to quivering of the ventricles, poor cardiac output, and death unless adequate ventricular function is established quickly. The ECG has irregular waves and it is difficult to identify any classic markings of the ECG (P waves, QRS, or T waves).

Long QT syndrome

LQTS is identified by delayed ventricular repolarization and seen as a prolongation of the corrected QT interval (QTc) on the ECG. This syndrome is a disorder of the ion channels causing a disruption in electrical impulse. The prevalence has been estimated as high as 1 in 2000 and can be inherited as an autosomal dominant or recessive trait.[24,25] LQTS syndrome has 2 forms, inherited or acquired. Thirteen different types of congenital LQTS have been found.[26] Acquired LQTS can be a result of medication administration or electrolyte imbalance. In some cases, the infant or person may have a mutation and an arrhythmia becomes apparent after a predisposing factor, such as a medication. This syndrome can cause an arrhythmia that spontaneously resolves but is also associated with an intermittent arrhythmia known as torsades de pointes. This arrhythmia is rapid and irregular and can develop into ventricular fibrillation and sudden death. LQTS is thought to be an implied contributor to 10% to 15% of sudden infant death syndrome (SIDS), and future research will focus on ECG screening to prevent these deaths.[24]

Sudden infant death syndrome

The incidence of SIDS in the United States is estimated to be 40 per 100,000 live births in 2013[27]; because SIDS is a sudden event, it is a diagnosis of exclusion. Importantly, NICU graduates are at higher risk for SIDS. Two major sources contributing to SIDS are infant sleep position[28] and dysfunctional cardiac sodium channels. Both acquired LQTS and the inherited (congenital) LQTS have been implicated in approximately 10% of SIDS cases.[29] LQTS puts the neonate at risk for sudden cardiac death.[12] It has components of bradycardia and tachycardia and is diagnosed by a prolonged QT interval on the ECG. Routine ECGs have not historically been performed but have been found feasible and accurate for cardiac monitoring in the NICU.[29] Monitors use algorithms to calculate baseline QTc and then continuously monitor to detect a variation.[30]

MECHANISMS OF ARRHYTHMIAS

Cardiac arrhythmias are either intrinsic or acquired. Intrinsic arrhythmias are either due to accessory pathways or SA node dysfunction, whereas acquired arrhythmias are due to electrolyte imbalance or medications.

Intrinsic Cardiac Arrhythmias

Accessory pathways

Accessory pathways are anomalous pieces of tissue formed during fetal development resulting in the initiation of extra electrical impulses or action potentials. An action potential is the electrical signal that is initiated and carries the impulse, which leads to the contraction of tissue. Accessory pathways can be either classic or concealed pathways.[20] In the classic pathway, the impulse travels from the atrium to the ventricles (antegrade), from the ventricles to the atrium (retrograde), or both (**Fig. 5**).

The classic pathway can be seen on the ECG as a delta wave caused by preexcitation during normal sinus rhythm (**Fig. 6**). Concealed pathways are not apparent on the ECG because there is no preexcitation and they only travel retrograde. A nodal or junctional rhythm occurs when the impulse originates near or at the AV node instead of the SA node. The heart rate is slower than the impulse originating at the SA node.[18]

Sinoatrial node dysfunction

The SA node is the primary pacemaker of the heart; *SA node dysfunction* is a general term that includes any condition leading to an inappropriately slow atrial rate. SA node dysfunction includes sinus bradycardia, junctional bradycardia, and

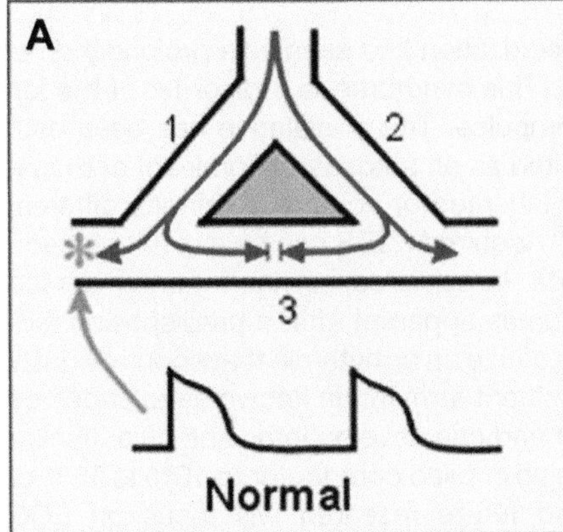

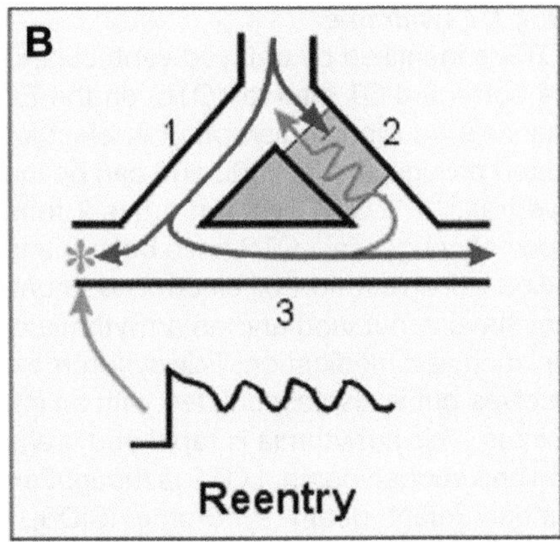

Fig. 5. Normal conduction of impulse (*A*) and reentry model (*B*). Panel A represents the normal impulse where 1 and 2 represent the action potential pathway from a single impulse; 3 is where the impulses meet and cancel each other out. Panel B represents the reentry model where the impulse is blocked at 2, so the impulse travels from 1 to 3 and back through 2 if the tissue is excitable instead of being canceled out and eliminated. The action potential shows the reduced velocity of the impulse related to the blocked impulse (*Asterisk* represents a single action potential in the location marked). (*From* Klabunde R. Cardiovascular physiology concepts. 2013. Available at: www.cvphysiology.com/Arrhythmias/A008c.htm. Accessed January 15, 2016; with permission.)

bradycardia-tachycardia syndrome; the rhythm remains regular unless bradycardia-tachycardia syndrome is present.[31] Cardiac surgery is the primary cause of SA node dysfunction.[32]

Acquired Cardiac Arrhythmias

Electrolyte imbalance

Hypokalemia and hyperkalemia can lead to arrhythmias. Hypokalemia can cause an increase in resting potential, which can lead to abnormal impulse formation and

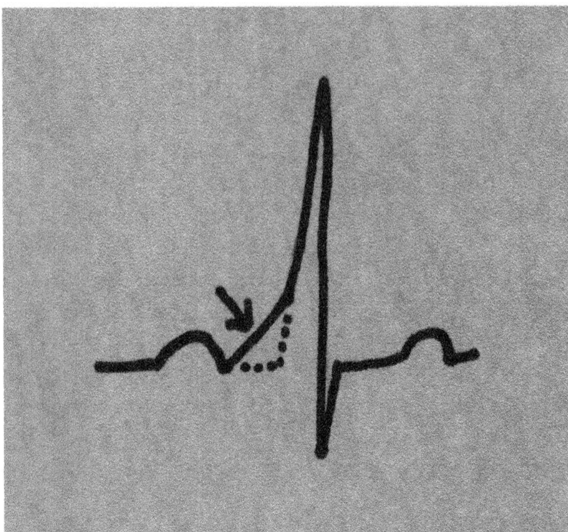

Fig. 6. The delta wave is evident on an ECG with shortened PR interval. The arrow indicates the curved or slurred onset of QRS complex. (*Courtesy of* Sherri L. McMullen, PhD, FNP, NNP-BC, Syracuse, NY.)

reentry arrhythmias.[33] Hyperkalemia can lead to decreased electrical conduction and a widened QRS complex, ventricular fibrillation, and asystole.[33,34] Magnesium, calcium, and sodium all impact the sodium-potassium pump and impact adequate functioning of the action potentials within the heart and body.[33] Hypermagnesium also can cause bradycardia.[35] Maintenance of normal electrolyte values optimizes cardiac function.

Medications

Proarrhythmia is a term used when a medication causes changes in the cardiac rhythm. These arrhythmias can affect conduction directly or indirectly through the autonomic nervous system or electrolyte disturbances. Medications, such as dopamine hydrochloride (a dopamine agonist at low doses), dobutamine (beta-1 agonist), and adrenaline (a beta-1 agonist at low doses), are catecholamines administered to improve contractility, cardiac output, and blood pressure but can lead to tachyarrhythmias.[36] Salbutamol or albuterol (a selective beta-2 adrenergic agonist) has been found to be associated with premature atrial contractions.[12] Some medications can indirectly cause arrhythmias by altering the electrolyte balance. Beta-adrenergic agonists can cause hypokalemia, which can lead to arrhythmias.[33] It is important for all who are prescribing and administering medications to be aware of the potential side effects, including electrolyte imbalances and potential changes in the heart rhythm.

TREATMENT OF NEONATAL ARRHYTHMIAS

If there is a suspicious ECG pattern on the bedside monitor or an infant is presenting in insidious and nonspecific ways with a suspected cardiac cause, a 12-lead ECG should be obtained. Diagnosis of a cardiac dysrhythmia depends on an experienced care provider to interpret this test. For some benign neonatal arrhythmias, observation with continued close assessment may be indicated, without further treatment. Binnetoglu and colleagues[37] found a good prognosis for infants with premature beats, with most of them disappearing within the first months of life. Infants diagnosed with congenital heart disease required additional attention when arrhythmias are present, and their clinical status must be monitored closely.

Treatment depends on the specific arrhythmia and the extent of hemodynamic compromise. Treatment can vary from observation to medication, transesophageal pacing, or cardioversion. There may be no treatment needed in the NICU for PACs, whereas treatment of SVT may be either digoxin or propranolol.[38] Treatment of other arrhythmias, such as atrial flutter, may require medical therapy with adenosine if transesophageal pacing is ineffective; if the infant is hemodynamically unstable, cardioversion may be necessary.[7] Infants with complete heart block, with a low heart rate (<50 beats per minute), and a wide QRS are usually symptomatic and would require an emergency pacemaker.[10] Treatment of LQTS with a beta-blocker has been found to reduce the risk of sudden death.[39] Treatment depends on the clinical status of patients and the type and cause of the arrhythmia.

NONCARDIAC APPLICATIONS FOR BEDSIDE CARDIAC MONITORING

Early Detection of Sepsis

Bedside cardiac monitoring technology has evolved over the last 50 years to recently provide bedside practitioners more than cardiac assessment. It can provide predictive monitoring to detect late-onset neonatal sepsis (LONS). LONS is identified by a positive blood culture obtained at 72 hours or greater after delivery and remains an important cause of infant morbidity and mortality.[40] The incidence is inversely proportionate to gestational age and birth weight with an incidence in 400 to 500 g infants as high as 65%.[41] Signs of LONS are nonspecific, and early detection of LONS is important to reduce morbidity and mortality.[40] In 2003, the US Food and Drug Administration approved the use of the HeRO monitor (Medical Predictive Science Corporation, Charlottesville, VA)[42]; as a result of the autonomic nervous system impact the sympathetic and parasympathetic systems have on beat-to-beat heart rate variability changes, subtle changes in heart rate can be detected.[43] Using specific data from heart rate R-R internal time series data and mathematical algorithms, the heart rate characteristics index score was developed and has been found to predict sepsis diagnosis within 24 hours.[40,43] There is no particular score that nurses need to alert supervising providers; instead, the nurse should note and report an increasing score.[42] The higher the heart rate characteristics index score, the higher the risk of diagnosis of LONS (with a score of 2 indicating a 2-fold increased risk, a score of 3 indicating a 3-fold increased risk, and so forth).[42] This score is considered in conjunction with other clinical assessments, and the clinical condition of the infant to determine if a septic workup and medical treatment is indicated. Importantly, using this heart rate characteristics and scoring system has been found to reduce infant mortality related to LONS by more than 20%.[44]

FUTURE RESEARCH

There is a great deal of future research needed in this area of neonatology. There is some discrepancy on reported incidence among many of the neonatal arrhythmias; in addition, the incidence and prevalence reported in publications are mostly more than 10 years old. With improvements in maternal and neonatal care, it is unclear if these earlier reported numbers remain relevant today. Further research in neonatal ECG monitoring is needed in this area as well as several additional areas. There are no guidelines regarding which NICU infants require cardiac bedside monitoring, so the standard practice is that all infants are continuously monitored until discharge. However, this practice of continuous monitoring is not based on research; parents may benefit from a transition period with the monitor off before discharge. Research is needed to determine if the 15-lead ECG offers utility in neonatal and infant populations. Further research is also needed to determine if screening for LQTS in infants and the NICU would save infant lives from sudden infant death.

SUMMARY

Electrocardiographic monitoring offers an incredible noninvasive strategy to identify potential complications in NICU patients. Recognition and examination of this information, either in isolation or in conjunction with additional data, can improve patient care. Technology continues to improve the care of our smallest and sickest patients; but there is no substitute for experienced human assessment and interpretation, and any concern about an arrhythmia should be reported so a referral to a pediatric cardiologist can be obtained. NICU nursing orientations should include specific information about what information cardiac monitoring offers and the importance of diligent observation of the bedside monitors. Orientation should also include the physiology behind the ECG changes on the bedside monitor and the importance of reporting these changes.

REFERENCES

1. Association of American Medical Colleges. Inside the neonatal intensive care unit: research advances care for hospitals' smallest patients. 2015. Available at: www.aamc.org/newsroom/reporter/january2015/422214/neonatal-care.html. Accessed December 18, 2015.
2. Centers for Disease Control and Prevention. Preterm birth. 2015. Available at: www.cdc.gov/reproductivehealth/maternalinfanthealth/pretermbirth.htm. Accessed December 20, 2015.
3. Centers for Disease Control and Prevention. Morbidity and mortality weekly report. 2013. Available at: www.cdc.gov/mmwr/preview/mmwrhtml/mm6231a3.htm. Accessed December 18, 2015.
4. Liebman J. The normal electrocardiogram in the newborn and neonatal period and its progression. J Electrocardiol 2010;43:524–9.
5. Fleming S, Thompson M, Stevens R, et al. Normal ranges of heart rate and respiratory rate in children from birth to 18 years: a systematic review of observational studies. Lancet 2011;377(9770):1011–8.
6. O'Connor M, McDaniel N, Brady WJ. The pediatric electrocardiogram: Part I: age related interpretation. Am J Emerg Med 2008;26:506–12.
7. Killen S, Fish F. Fetal and neonatal arrhythmias. NeoReviews 2008;9(6):e242–52.
8. Schwartz P, Garson A, Paul T, et al. Guidelines for the interpretation of the neonatal electrocardiogram. Eur Heart J 2002;23:1329–44.
9. Attallah L, Serteyn A, Meftah M, et al. Unobtrusive ECG monitoring in the NICU using a capacitive sensing array. Physiol Meas 2014;35:895–913.
10. Dublin A. Arrhythmias in the newborn. NeoReviews 2000;1(8):146–51.
11. Turner C, Wren C. The epidemiology of arrhythmias in infants: a population-based study. J Paediatr Child Health 2013;49:278–81.
12. Badrawi N, Hegazy R, Tikovic E, et al. Arrhythmia in the neonatal intensive care unit. Pediatr Cardiol 2009;30:325–30.
13. Davignon A, Rautaharju P, Boisselle E, et al. Normal ECG standards for infants and children. Pediatr Cardiol 1980;1:123–52.
14. Artman M, Mahony L, Teitel D. Neonatal cardiology. New York: McGraw-Hill; 2010.
15. Eichenwald E. Apnea of prematurity. Pediatrics 2016;137(1):e1–7.
16. Fillips D, Bucciarelli R. Cardiac evaluation of the newborn. Pediatr Clin North Am 2015;62:471–89.
17. Strasburger J, Cheulkar B, Wichman H. Perinatal arrhythmias: diagnosis and management. Clin Perinatol 2007;34(4):627–52.
18. Isik D, Celik I, Kavurt S, et al. A case series of neonatal arrhythmias. J Matern Fetal Neonatal Med 2016;29(8):1344–7. Available at: www.tandfonline.com/doi/full/10.3109/14767058.2015.1048679. Accessed December 18, 2015.
19. Hornik C, Chu P, Li J, et al. Comparative effectiveness of digoxin and propranolol for supraventricular tachycardia in infants. Pediatr Crit Care Med 2014;15(9):839–45.
20. Hermosura T, Bradshaw W. Wolf-Parkinson-White syndrome in infants. Neonatal Netw 2010;29(4):215–23.
21. Klabunde R. Cardiovascular physiology concepts. 2013. Available at: www.cvphysiology.com/Arrhythmias/A008c.htm. Accessed January 15, 2016.
22. Goldhill D, Latosa E. Anesthesia and Wolff-Parkinson-White syndrome during infancy: a review. J R Soc Med 1988;81(81):345–7.
23. Valderrama A. Essentials for the primary care nurse practitioner. J Am Acad Nurse Pract 2004;16:378–83.

24. Schwartz PJ, Stramba-Badiale M, Crotti L, et al. Prevalence of the congenital long-QT syndrome. Circulation 2009;120:1761–7.
25. Tester D, Ackerman M. Cardiomyopathic and channelopathic causes of sudden infant death in infants and children. Annu Rev Med 2009;60:69–84.
26. Ackerman M, Priori S, Willems S, et al. HRS/EHRA expert consensus statement on the state of genetic testing for the channelopathies and cardiomyopathies. Heart Rhythm 2011;8(8):1308–39.
27. Mathews T, MacDorman M, Thoma M. Infant mortality statistics from the 2013 period linked birth/infant death data set. Natl Vital Stat Rep 2015;64(9):1–30. Available at: http://www.cdc.gov/nchs/data/nvsr/nvsr64/nvsr64_09.pdf.
28. McMullen S. Transitioning premature infants supine: state of the science. MCN Am J Matern Child Nurs 2016;38(1):8–12.
29. Helfenbein ED, Ackerman MJ, Rautaharju PM, et al. An algorithm for QT monitoring in neonatal intensive care units. J Electrocardiol 2007;40(6):S103–10.
30. Helfenbein E, Zhou S, Lindauer J, et al. An algorithm for continuous real-time QT interval monitoring. J Electrocardiol 2006;39:S123–7.
31. Zeigler V. Pediatric cardiac arrhythmias resulting in hemodynamic compromise. Crit Care Nurs Clin North Am 2005;17:77–95.
32. LeRoy S, Dick M. Practical managment of pediatric cardiac arrhythmias. New York: Futura Publishing; 2001.
33. Barnes B, Holland J. Drug-induced arrhythmias. Crit Care Med 2010;38(6): S188–97.
34. Weisberg LS. Management of severe hyperkalemia. Crit Care Med 2008;36: 3246–51.
35. Hyun H, Choi H, Kim J, et al. Idiopathic severe hypermagnesemia in an extremely low birth weight infant on the first day of life. Korean J Pediatr 2011;54(7):310–2.
36. Benham-Hermetz J, Lambert M, Stephens R. Cardiovascular failure, inotropes and vasopressors. Br J Hosp Med 2012;73(5):C74–7. Available at: https://www.ucl.ac.uk/anaesthesia/StudentsandTrainees/Inotropes_Vasopressors.
37. Binnetoglu F, Baboglu K, Altun G, et al. Diagnosis, treatment and follow up of neonatal arrhythmias. Cardiovasc J Afr 2014;25(2):58–62.
38. Sanatani S, Potts J, Reed J, et al. The study of antiarrhythmic medications in infancy (SAMIS). Circ Arrhythm Electrophysiol 2012;5:984–91.
39. Kopponen M, Marjamaa A, Hiippala A, et al. Follow-up of 316 molecularly defined pediatric long-QT syndrome patients: clinical course, treatments and side effects. Circ Arrhythm Electrophysiol 2015;8:815–23.
40. Fairchild K. Predictive monitoring for early detection of sepsis in neonatal ICU patients. Curr Opin Pediatr 2013;25(2):172–9.
41. Dong Y, Speer C. Late-onset neonatal sepsis: recent developments. Arch Dis Child Fetal Neonatal Ed 2015;100:F257–63.
42. Hicks J, Fairchild K. Heart rate characteristics in the NICU. Adv Neonatal Care 2013;13(6):396–401.
43. Fairchild KD, O'Shea TM. Heart rate characteristics: physiomarkers for detection of late-onset neonatal sepsis. Clin Perinatol 2010;37(3):581–98.
44. Moorman JR, Carlo WA, Kattwinkel J, et al. Mortality reduction by heart rate characteristic monitoring in very low birth weight neonates: a randomized trial. J Pediatr 2011;159:900–6.

In-Hospital Cardiac Arrest

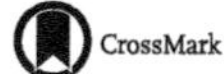

An Update on Pulseless Electrical Activity and Asystole

Mina Attin, PhD, RN*, Rebecca G. Tucker, PhD, ACNPC, MEd, RN,
Mary G. Carey, PhD, RN

KEYWORDS

- In-hospital cardiac arrest • Pulseless electrical activity • Asystole
- Cardiac arrhythmia • Resuscitation

KEY POINTS

- Common cardiac arrhythmias preceding in-hospital cardiac arrest are pulseless electrical activity and asystole, known as nonshockable rhythms.
- In the hospital, nurses are often the first witnesses of and responders to cardiac arrest and they immediately must initiate high-quality cardiopulmonary resuscitation.
- Timely and high-quality cardiopulmonary resuscitation is the primary treatment for non-shockable rhythms, not defibrillation.
- Further research in all aspects of nonshockable rhythms is recommended due to the disparity in scientific information and higher morbidity and mortality when compared to shockable rhythms, including ventricular tachycardia and ventricular fibrillation.

INTRODUCTION

Cardiac arrest (CA) is a significant public health problem with catastrophic consequences for the survivors, their families, and the health care system. It is categorized as out-of-hospital cardiac arrest (O-HCA) or in-hospital cardiac arrest (I-HCA). Cardiac arrhythmias, specifically shockable rhythms, including pulseless ventricular tachycardia (VT) and ventricular fibrillation (VF), have been identified as one of the major causes of O-HCA. Recent studies have reported varying incidences and prevalences of VT/VF, yet nonshockable rhythms are being reported more often in both O-HCA and I-HCA. Nonshockable rhythms include pulseless electrical activity (PEA) and asystole. This emerging change of cardiac arrhythmias preceding CA is due to a variety of factors that may encompass demographics, pathophysiology, and advances in therapeutic treatments.[1–6]

Disclosure Statement: None of the authors have any conflicts to disclose.
University of Rochester School of Nursing, 601 Elmwood Avenue, BOX SON, Rochester, NY 14642, USA
* Corresponding author.
E-mail address: Mina_Attin@urmc.rochester.edu

Crit Care Nurs Clin N Am 28 (2016) 387–397
http://dx.doi.org/10.1016/j.cnc.2016.04.010 **ccnursing.theclinics.com**
0899-5885/16/$ – see front matter © 2016 Elsevier Inc. All rights reserved.

The American Heart Association (AHA) has launched a national registry known as Get with The Guidelines-Resuscitation (GWTG-R), formerly known as National Registry of Cardiopulmonary Resuscitation (NRCPR) that collects and analyzes data on adult and pediatric I-HCA from approximately 10% of hospitals in the United States. By so doing, it has identified quality improvement opportunities and has provided performance comparisons among participating hospitals. Numerous published studies using data from this national registry have improved our understanding of I-HCA and have improved the quality of care at hospitals. Important published findings, including those reporting that there is a lower rate of survival of I-HCA during nights and weekends and that the time of defibrillation during CA should be less than or equal to 2 minutes, are examples of such studies and testify to the value of this AHA-initiated program.[5]

It has been acknowledged by national organizations that I-HCA has not received the same attention as O-HCA. Consequently, there are many gaps in the knowledge and science concerning the optimal way of providing effective care.[2,3] Thus, the purpose of the present article is to provide an overview of nonshockable cardiac arrhythmias preceding I-HCA, specifically PEA and asystole, and to discuss nursing's role in the application of science to practice.

DEFINITIONS

Pseudo-Pulseless Electrical Activity and True Pulseless Electrical Activity

Historically, PEA has been defined as the dissociation between the electrical and mechanical activity of the heart. The electrical depolarization occurs with no synchronous cardiac myocyte shortening. More recent definitions of PEA refer to syndromes characterized by the presence of the heart's electrical activity, excluding ventricular tachyarrhythmias with no palpable pulse. According to this definition, the presence of any rhythm or arrhythmia except tachyarrhythmias originating in the ventricles with no pulse can be defined as PEA.[2,7]

A phenomenon that is called pseudo-PEA refers to the presence of electrical activity with very weak myocardial contraction that is not able to generate a pulse, common in conditions such as in severe shock. It precedes true PEA and the survival rate of patients is higher than for those suffering true PEA on implementation of therapeutic interventions.[7] One of the most common initial rhythms that precede I-HCA is PEA. A diagnosis of pseudo-PEA requires the confirmation of weak myocardial contraction by certain equipment (eg, echocardiography) that is not usually performed during the busy time of resuscitation. An example of electrocardiographic (ECG) characteristics during pseudo-PEA may include a narrow QRS complex tachycardia as opposed to the wide QRS complex bradyarrhythmias that may be present during true PEA.[7]

Asystole

Asystole refers to a state in which there is no electrical and mechanical activity of the heart. Asystole is usually assumed to be a consequence of untreated or unsuccessful treatment of such cardiac arrhythmias as VT/VF. Another common term that is used by clinicians/scientists instead of asystole is bradyasystole, defined as a cardiac rhythm with a ventricular rate below 60 beats per minute with periods of asystole (no heart rhythm).[8] Bradyasystole is also defined as sinus node arrest or atrioventricular node block with asystole or a slow escape rhythm, 30 beats per minute.[9] Bradycardia with or without pulse occurs in CA as an initial rhythm either during resuscitation or after electrical defibrillation.[10] Asystole occurs in all dying patients.[10]

In-Hospital Cardiac Arrest

I-HCA is defined as a state of apnea and unresponsiveness accompanied by the absence of a palpable central pulse in patients without do not resuscitate (DNR) orders and who received cardiopulmonary resuscitation (CPR).[3]

PROFESSIONAL ORGANIZATIONS COMMIT TO IMPROVE SURVIVAL RATES IN CARDIAC ARRESTS

In 2010, the Emergency Cardiovascular Care Committee of the AHA set a 2020 goal of doubling the rate of survival of both O-HCA and I-HCA, from 19% to 38%.[11] In 2013, the AHA released a consensus statement entitled "Strategies for Improving Survival after In-Hospital CA in the United States."[3] The statement begins with the operational definition of I-HCA as the number of patients who receive chest compressions, defibrillation, or both (regardless of admission status); any patient with O-HCA should not be included and all patients with a DNR order before or ordered during mid-arrest should not be included. With regard to outcomes, the minimum standard is survival to hospital discharge, but survival to 30 days along with a measure of functional status is preferred. Best practices were described in 3 stages: pre-arrest, intra-arrest, and post-arrest. When discussing pre–I-HCA, an emphasis on access to defibrillation within 2 minutes plus the presence of standardized equipment throughout the hospital was emphasized. Two types of response teams were called for: a rapid response team (about whose effectiveness current data are mixed)[12,13] and the code teams that are required by the Joint Commission.[14] In addition, the 2004 AHA Scientific Statement[15] says that O-HCA patients resuscitated from CA benefit from cardiac monitoring for at least 48 hours after admission. In looking at intra-arrest, it has been shown that high-quality chest compression improves outcomes among I-HCA survivors.[16,17] Almost half of the occurrences of I-HCA are outside of the intensive care unit (ICU)[18]; thus, implementation of automatic external defibrillators outside of ICUs may improve resuscitation success rates.[19] Concerns after arrest include brain injury, myocardial dysfunction, systemic ischemia, or reperfusion response, and persistent pathology that precipitated the I-HCA. Importantly, the consensus statement highlights the importance of changing the perception that I-HCA survival is hopeless. This consensus statement ends with institutional recommendations that are focused on establishing and implementing the best practices, such as reporting patient self-determination and implementing a standardized, evidence-based prognostication approach to prevent premature withdrawal of life-sustaining therapy.[3]

The Institute of Medicine (IOM) of the National Academies serves as an independent and objective national advisor for the improvement of the population's health. In 2015, the IOM published a report titled "Strategies to Improve "Cardiac Arrest Survival: A Time to Act."[4] CA was described as a severe malfunction or cessation of the electrical and mechanical activity of the heart resulting in almost instantaneous loss of consciousness and collapse. Eight strategies were recommended for improving CA survival:

1. Establish a national CA registry
2. Foster a culture of action through public awareness and training
3. Enhance the capabilities and performance of emergency medical services systems
4. Set national accreditation standards related to CA for hospitals and health care systems
5. Adopt continuous quality improvement programs
6. Accelerate research on pathophysiology, new therapies, and translation of science for CA

7. Accelerate research on the evaluation and adoption of CA therapies
8. Create a national CA collaborative

In response, the AHA released a special report[5] announcing 4 new commitments to improve CA survival. The AHA committed itself to (1) providing up to $5 million in funding over 5 years to incentivize resuscitation data interoperability; (2) pursuing philanthropic support for improving out- and in-hospital systems of care so as to increase cardiac arrest survival; (3) seeking philanthropic support for launching a resuscitation research network; and (4) sponsoring a National Cardiac Arrest Summit as a means of facilitating a national collaboration on the subject of cardiac arrest. Both the AHA and the IOM have recommended future studies to address the gap between science and practice so as to improve overall survival rate after I-HCA.

EPIDEMIOLOGY OF PULSELESS ELECTRICAL ACTIVITY AND ASYSTOLE

Incidence

I-HCA constitutes a significant public health problem, accounting for approximately 200,000 treated CAs annually in the United States.[20] It is estimated that approximately half of treated I-HCA consists of avoidable arrest.[21] This includes arrest preceded by delays in response to changes in vital signs and delays in the activation of medical personnel.[3,21] The presence of 3 critically abnormal vital signs has been associated with high mortality.[22]

Trends of Cardiac Arrhythmias

I-HCA studies using registry data from GWTG-R have reported a high incidence of PEA and asystole in comparison with VT and VF; greater than 70% of initial rhythms are non-VT/VF.[23] One study, published in 2003, reported the incidence of VT and VF as the first documented rhythm for I-HCA as 25%, whereas the incidence of asystole and PEA were 36% and 30%, respectively.[18] The proportion of PEA and asystole before I-HCA recently has been reported to have increased from 69% to 84% in the years between 2000 and 2009.[1]

The increase in PEA and asystole has been speculated to be related to different factors,[6] including the decreased death due to acute myocardial infarction leading to a decreased sudden cardiac death,[24] the advancement of interventions such as defibrillation for treating VT/VF, an aging population, the presence of chronic illness, and certain medications, including antipsychotic medications and possibly beta blockers.[2,24] However, the exact underlying mechanisms are still unknown.[2]

Survival Rates

The overall initial survival rate (with survival being defined as the return of spontaneous circulation) of patients with asystole and PEA is much lower than the survival rate for patients who experienced pulseless VT or VF (35% and 39% vs 63% and 58%, respectively).[18] The overall rate of survival to hospital discharge of I-HCA remains low, although it has recently improved from approximately 15% to 20%. The most recent statistics (2013) show an improvement in overall survival to hospital discharge (24%).[1,25] A wide, variable survival rate has been reported from different types of hospitals (eg, academic and nonacademic hospitals), yet recent statistics could not explain the differences by the patient case-mix or hospital characteristics.[26] Further research is needed to investigate the crucial factors influencing the survival rates.

Locations

I-HCA studies have shown that approximately 50% of I-HCAs occur within the ICU.[27,28] Other units in which I-HCA occurs are telemetry or nontelemetry units (15% in each type of unit) and the rest take place in the emergency room or any other location at hospitals. This shows that I-HCA could occur anywhere at hospitals.[25] A multicenter study showed that only 16% of the ICU population survived to discharge after receiving CPR therapy.[27] Most I-HCA research that is focused on ICU settings is limited to single center studies that demonstrate widely varied results, probably due to varying population characteristics. Moreover, the highest rates of survival to hospital discharge (60%–79%) have been reported by surgical ICUs.[29]

Short-Term and Long-Term Outcomes

One of the major complications for CA survivors is neurologic deficits. One common and well-established tool for evaluating the neurologic damage is the cerebral performance category (CPC), which ranges from CPC1 (return to normal cerebral performance) to CPC 5 (brain death). A recent study[30] investigated the extent of neurologic deficit among CA survivors who had CPC 1 or 2. Impairment of long-term memory with intact short-term memory was the major neurologic deficit among these patients. Another major complication afflicting survivors of CA is congestive heart failure, which has been found to be responsible for a high readmission rate for I-HCA survivors.[31]

NONSHOCKABLE RHYTHMS IN CARDIAC AND NONCARDIAC DISEASES

Traditionally, nonshockable rhythms have been attributed to a variety of reversible conditions, frequently remembered using the mnemonic device "4H4T." The "4H4T" stands for Hypoxia, Hypovolemia, Hypo/Hyperkalemia, Hypothermia; Thrombosis/Pulmonary Emboli, Tamponade Cardiac, Toxins, and Tension pneumothorax. Other pathologies that are not included in the "4H4T" have been identified as causes of PEA arrest, including cardiac diseases[32–34] and sepsis. Recent limited reports[33,34] have shown that cardiac disease accounts for at least 50% of all occurrences of I-HCA and that the initial rhythms of PEA and asystole are not strictly of noncardiac origin. Yet the exact cause of I-HCA, the determination of which is necessary for discovering appropriate treatments, is often missed.

A landmark study[35] in 1989 revealed that the cause of sudden death in patients with advanced heart failure (New York Heart Association Class III or IV heart failure) was multifactorial. These patients with heart failure were monitored by ECG telemetry systems during their hospitalizations and their initial rhythms of CA were identified as VT/VF, bradyarrhythmias, and PEA. Another study[36] in 2005 showed asystole and PEA as the initial rhythms of CA among patients with orthotopic heart transplantation, most of whom (82%) died in an inpatient setting.

It has been suggested that diagnostic ECG clues in conjunction with a patient's history and examination can be used to identify the underlying etiology and predict the likelihood of survival.[7] For example, PEA with rapid heart rate can be due to hypovolemia or tension pneumothorax, rather than metabolic or electrolyte imbalances. However, CAs are very chaotic times and clinicians may not pay attention to rhythms of PEA. Telemetry has been recognized as an independent predictor of survival to hospital discharge in non–critical care patients who experience I-HCA (**Fig. 1**).[37] Recent studies have focused on studying the telemetry to investigate the retrospective patterns of diagnostic ECG clues. Cardiac arrhythmias, specifically bradycardia, have been identified as independent predictors of mortality among patients who suffer

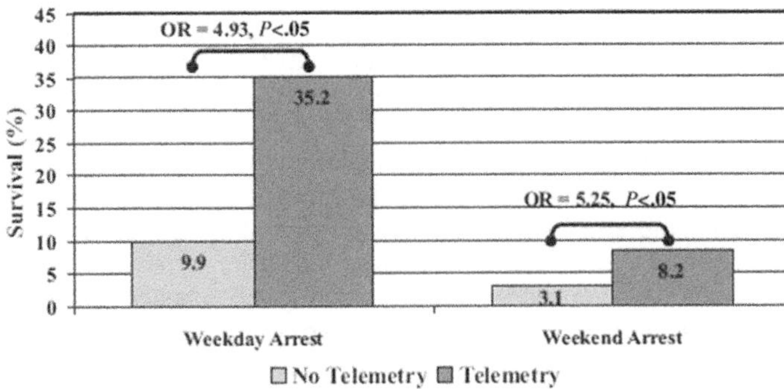

Fig. 1. Survival rate of the initial cardiac arrest stratified by day of week and use of telemetry. (*From* Cleverley K, Mousavi N, Stronger L, et al. The impact of telemetry on survival of in-hospital cardiac arrests in non-critical care patients. Resuscitation 2013;84(7):880; with permission.)

I-HCA.[38] Thus, continuous cardiac monitoring during hospitalization is important insofar as it may indicate the genesis of the mechanism of cardiac arrhythmias.[9,39]

NURSING PERSPECTIVE

Most nursing literature has focused on describing and studying VT/VF, the classic rhythms of cardiac arrest. It has not devoted adequate attention to I-HCA, particularly with respect in PEA and asystole. High-quality and timely CPR should be emphasized for patients who suffer PEA and asystole, just as timely defibrillation is emphasized for patients who experience VT/VF. Poor application of knowledge and skills during resuscitation has resulted in patient mortality,[40] and delayed administration of vasopressors (>5 minutes, time interval between CA and the first dose) has been linked to decreased survival after I-HCA.[23] Addressing errors during resuscitation is as important as identifying patients at risk of CA due to PEA and asystole, insofar as both of these factors influence the rate of survival.

Nurses, working within an interdisciplinary team, can have a significant impact on preventing or minimizing the catastrophic consequences of I-HCA. However, it has been documented that nurses often do not have time to be part of an interdisciplinary team, a situation that has been categorized as "missed care."[41] The prevention of CA can be achieved partly by detecting early signs of deterioration (**Fig. 2**). However, detection of early signs and effective resuscitation therapy during CA by nurses are influenced by various factors, such as work environment, resources, and value systems.

Work Environment and Nursing Staffing

It is well documented that inadequate registered nurse (RN) staffing and poor working environment influence patients' complications and mortality.[42,43] The National Institute of Nursing Research has acknowledged the importance of studying the relationship between nursing staffing and mortality as one of the 10 landmark studies that impact nursing practice and patient lives.[44] Even the most competent nurse may commit preventable errors when taxed with a daily work load that exceeds a reasonable assignment. The high mortality rate of PEA and asystole requires an interdisciplinary team at bedside to prevent complications and potential CA. To function effectively as part of such an interdisciplinary team, nurses must have adequate support and a

I knew it was coming.
Call a code blue!!!
Hypovolemia
Cardiac Tamponade
Acidosis
Pulmonary Embolism
Code Blue
No Oxygen
No Circulation
Hypoglycemia
Myocardial Infarction
Drug Overdose
Sepsis
Tension Pneumothorax
Electrolyte Imbalance
Not on my shift!
Mr. Smith, I'm going
to check your vital signs again.
How are you feeling?
I don't feel well.
But I don't know what's
wrong with me.
Missing early signs of deterioration prior to I-HCA
Monitoring for early signs of deterioration prior to I-HCA

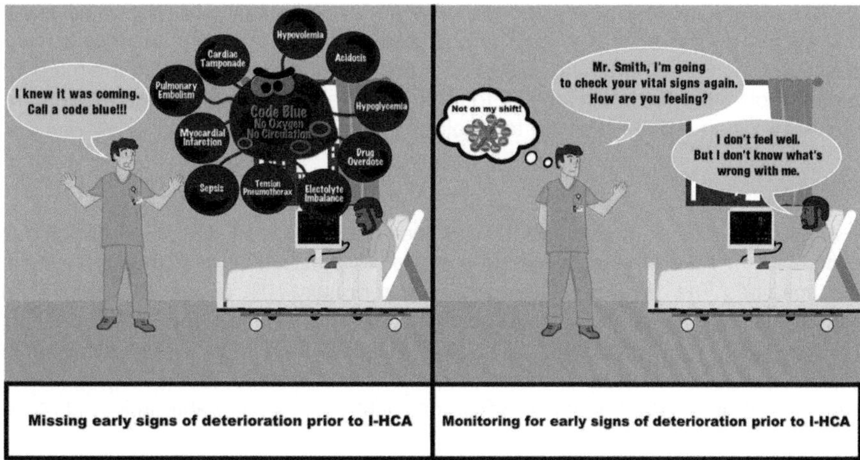

Fig. 2. The importance of monitoring for deteriorating early signs of I-HCA by a nurse. (*Courtesy of* Mina Attin, PhD, Rebecca G. Tucker, PhD, and Mary G. Carey, PhD. Copyright © 2016; used with permission of Mina Attin, PhD, University of Rochester School of Nursing, Rochester, NY.)

reasonable work load. Knowledge of pathophysiology, resuscitation, and underlying causes of CA cannot be translated into nursing interventions when one's work load or/and work environment is beyond an individual's capacity. Moreover, it has been demonstrated[21] that the survival rate of I-HCA is lower during nights and weekends, even after adjusting for patient, event, and hospital characteristics. It has been speculated that this pattern may be related to inadequate staffing and available resources (diagnostic tests), insofar as nights and weekends are concerned; also, these are the times in which staff numbers systematically diminish. Nursing literature has documented these characteristics of staffing and resources during weekend and night shifts.[45,46]

Resources

Frequent educational programs (eg, simulated CAs for nurses, MOCK code blue) are necessary for nurses to maintain their competencies (including resuscitation skills) and knowledge that, otherwise, has been demonstrated to quickly deteriorate after 3 months.[47] The AHA still requires advanced cardiac life support certification to be renewed only every 2 years. Furthermore, the frequency with which a hospital can conduct competency sessions (eg, MOCK code blue) using simulated CA scenarios is limited due to their cost and the demands of staffing in a given hospital. One solution to the problems is found in the utilization of technology, including online recertifications and simulation laboratories that can mimic CA scenarios that have already occurred in a given hospital. Nurses thereby can learn how to prevent making the same mistake either before or during resuscitation.

Training

It is well known that I-HCA occurs in situations in which recognized signs of deterioration do not prompt clinicians to take action to activate a rapid response team (RRT). Recently, a study[48] reported that the most common reason for a failure to activate the RRT is the clinician's own perception of having control over the situation in a hospital setting in which patients require a higher level of care. Another important aspect is the quality of education of nursing students. Training a new generation of nursing students who are accustomed to technology should be part of the solution to I-HCA. Examining and analyzing retrospective clinical data must be an acquired value system for nursing students before graduation. Additionally, the health care industry and nurses in particular should prioritize collating and presenting the massive amount of physiologic data available to them into presentable and interpretable conclusions by using rapidly evolving technology.

SUMMARY

Most I-HCA studies are published through the national registry, GWTG-R, which has significantly improved the understanding of the magnitude and multidimensionality of CA at hospitals. The data from this registry only represent 10% of hospitals across the United States and these hospitals volunteer to share CA data with the AHA. A national registry documenting CA is crucial to a fuller understanding of the mechanism of CA and the improvement of treatment and prevention. Furthermore, the underlying mechanism should be interpreted in light of gender differences due to anatomic and physiologic differences between men and women.[49,50]

Nurses have a pivotal role in managing the lethal cardiac arrhythmias that lead to I-HCA. As the first responders to I-HCA, nurses must have the proper knowledge and training to provide timely and efficient CPR therapy. Due to the increasing prevalence of I-HCA with initial rhythms of PEA and asystole, there is an increased need for additional training of bedside nurses to enable them to quickly and accurately interpret ECGs. More nursing research is needed to further understand the phenomena of PEA and asystole, enhance treatment options, and provide education to nurses.

ACKNOWLEDGMENTS

We thank Dr Ying Xue, DNSc, RN, associate professor in the School of Nursing, for her critical review of the article, and to Joseph Gomulak-Cavicchio, MSED, and Philip R. Frey for their assistance in making the "early deterioration signs" cartoon.

REFERENCES

1. Girotra S, Nallamothu BK, Spertus JA, et al, American Heart Association Get with the Guidelines–Resuscitation (GWTG Resuscitation) Investigators. Trends in survival after in-hospital cardiac arrest. N Engl J Med 2012;367(20):1912–20.
2. Myerburg RJ, Halperin H, Egan DA, et al. Pulseless electric activity, definition, causes, mechanisms, management, and research priorities for the next decade: report from a National Heart, Lung, and Blood Institute Workshop. Circulation 2013;128(23):2532–41.
3. Morrison LJ, Neumar RW, Zimmerman JL, et al, American Heart Association Emergency Cardiovascular Care Committee, Council on Cardiopulmonary Critical Care, Perioperative and Resuscitation. Strategies for improving survival after in-hospital cardiac arrest in the United States: 2013 consensus recommendations: a consensus statement from the American Heart Association. Circulation 2013;127(14):1538–63.
4. Graham R, McCoy MA, Schultz AM. Strategies to improve cardiac arrest survival: a time to act. Washington, DC: National Academies Press (US); 2015.
5. Neumar RW, Eigel B, Callaway CW, et al. American Heart Association Response to the 2015 Institute of Medicine Report on Strategies to Improve Cardiac Arrest Survival. Circulation 2015;132(11):1049–70.
6. Goldberger J, Basu A, Boineau R, et al. Risk stratification for sudden cardiac death: a plan for the future. Circulation 2014;129(4):516–26.

7. Mehta C, Brady W. Pulseless electrical activity in cardiac arrest: electrocardiographic presentations and management considerations based on the electrocardiogram. Am J Emerg Med 2012;30(1):236–9.
8. Cady CE, Aufderheide TP. Etiology, electrophysiology, myocardial energy mechanics, and treatment of bradyasystole. In: Ornato JP, Peberdy MA, editors. Cardiopulmonary resuscitation. Totowa (NJ): Springer Science & Business Media; 2007. p. 123–30.
9. Do DH, Hayase J, Tiecher RD, et al. ECG changes on continuous telemetry preceding in-hospital cardiac arrests. J Electrocardiol 2015;48(6):1062–8.
10. Ornato JP, Peberdy MA. The mystery of bradyasystole during cardiac arrest. Ann Emerg Med 1996;27(5):576–87.
11. Association AH. Emergency cardiovascular care 2020 impact goals. 2010. Available at: http://www.heart.org/HEARTORG/General/Emergency-Cardiovascular-Care-2020-Impact-Goals_UCM_435128_Article.jsp#. Accessed March 30, 2016.
12. Bellomo R, Goldsmith D, Uchino S, et al. A prospective before-and-after trial of a medical emergency team. Med J Aust 2003;179(6):283–7.
13. Hillman K, Chen J, Cretikos M, et al. Introduction of the medical emergency team (MET) system: a cluster-randomized controlled trial. Lancet 2005;365(9477): 2091–7.
14. Commission TJ. Commission-Requirements Hospitals. 2013. Available at: https://www.jointcommission.org/standards_information/tjc_requirements.aspx. Accessed March 30, 2016.
15. Drew BJ, Califf RM, Funk M, et al. Practice standards for electrocardiographic monitoring in hospital settings: an American Heart Association Scientific Statement from the Councils on Cardiovascular Nursing, Clinical Cardiology, and Cardiovascular Disease in the Young: endorsed by the International Society of Computerized Electrocardiology and the American Association of Critical-Care Nurses. Circulation 2004;110(17):2721–46.
16. Abella BS, Sandbo N, Vassilatos P, et al. Chest compression rates during cardiopulmonary resuscitation are suboptimal: a prospective study during in-hospital cardiac arrest. Circulation 2005;111(4):428–34.
17. Abella BS, Alvarado JP, Myklebust H, et al. Quality of cardiopulmonary resuscitation during in-hospital cardiac arrest. JAMA 2005;293(3):305–10.
18. Peberdy MA, Kaye W, Ornato JP, et al. Cardiopulmonary resuscitation of adults in the hospital: a report of 14720 cardiac arrests from the National Registry of Cardiopulmonary Resuscitation. Resuscitation 2003;58(3):297–308.
19. Gombotz H, Weh B, Mitterndorfer W, et al. In-hospital cardiac resuscitation outside the ICU by nursing staff equipped with automated external defibrillators—the first 500 cases. Resuscitation 2006;70(3):416–22.
20. Peng TJ, Anderson LW, Saindon BZ, et al. The administration of dextrose during in-hospital cardiac arrest is associated with increased mortality and neurologic morbidity. Crit Care 2015;19(1):160.
21. Peberdy MA, Ornato JP, Larkin GL, et al. National Registry of Cardiopulmonary Resuscitation Investigators. survival from in-hospital cardiac arrest during nights and weekends. JAMA 2008;299(7):785–92.
22. Bleyera AJ, Vidyab S, Russellb GB, et al. Longitudinal analysis of one million vital signs in patients in an academic medical center. Resuscitation 2011;82(11): 1387–92.
23. Ornato JP, Peberdy MA, Reid RD, et al, NRCPR Investigators. Impact of resuscitation system errors on survival from in-hospital cardiac arrest. Resuscitation 2012;83(1):63–9.

24. Dalen JE, Alpert JS, Goldberg RJ, et al. The epidemic of the 20th century: coronary heart disease. Am J Med 2014;127(9):807–12.
25. Chan PS. Public health burden of in-hospital cardiac arrest. Commissioned by the Institute of Medicine Committee on Treatment of Cardiac Arrest: current status and future directions. 2015. Available at: https://www.nationalacademies.org/hmd/~/media/Files/Report%20Files/2015/GWTG.pdf. Accessed March 30, 2016.
26. Merchant RM, Berg RA, Yang L, et al. Hospital variation in survival after in-hospital cardiac arrest. J Am Heart Assoc 2014;3(1):e000400.
27. Tian J, Kaufman DA, Zarich S, et al. Outcomes of critically ill patients who received cardiopulmonary resuscitation. Am J Respir Crit Care Med 2010;182(4):501–6.
28. Khan AM, Kirkpatrick JN, Yang L, et al. Age, sex, and hospital factors are associated with the duration of cardiopulmonary resuscitation in hospitalized patients who do not experience sustained return of spontaneous circulation. J Am Heart Assoc 2014;3(6):e001044.
29. Efendijev I, Nurmi J, Castren M, et al. Incidence and outcome from adult cardiac arrest occurring in the intensive care units: a systematic review of the literature. Resuscitation 2014;85(4):472–9.
30. Sulzgrubera P, Kliegel A, Wandallera C, et al. Survivors of cardiac arrest with good neurological outcome show considerable impairments of memory functioning. Resuscitation 2015;88:120–5.
31. Chan PS, Nallamothu BK, Krumholz HM, et al. Readmission rates and long-term hospital costs among survivors of an in-hospital cardiac arrest. Circ Cardiovasc Qual Outcomes 2014;7(6):889–95.
32. Beun L, Yersin B, Osterwalder J, et al. Pulseless electrical activity cardiac arrest: time to amend the mnemonic "4H&4T"? Swiss Med Wkly 2015;145:w14178.
33. Saarinen S, Nurmi J, Toivio T, et al. Does appropriate treatment of the primary underlying cause of PEA during resuscitation improve patients' survival? Resuscitation 2012;83(7):819–22.
34. Wallmuller C, Meron G, Kurkciyan I, et al. Causes of in-hospital cardiac arrest and influence on outcome. Resuscitation 2012;83(10):1206–11.
35. Luu M, Stevenson WG, Stevenson LW, et al. Diverse mechanisms of unexpected cardiac arrest in advanced heart failure. Circulation 1989;80:1675–80.
36. Vaseghi M, Lellouche N, Ritter H, et al. Mode and mechanisms of death following orthotopic heart transplantation. Heart Rhythm 2009;6(4):503–9.
37. Cleverley K, Mousavi N, Stronger L, et al. The impact of telemetry on survival of in-hospital cardiac arrests in non-critical care patients. Resuscitation 2013;84(7):878–82.
38. Bhalala US, Bonafide CP, Coletti C, et al. Antecedent bradycardia and in-hospital cardiopulmonary arrest mortality in telemetry-monitored patients outside the ICU. Resuscitation 2012;83(9):1106–10.
39. Attin M, Feld G, Wang L, et al. Electrocardiogram characteristics prior to in-hospital cardiac arrest. J Clin Monit Comput 2015;29(3):385–92.
40. Panesar SS, Ignatowicz AM, Donaldson LJ. Errors in the management of cardiac arrest: an observational study of patient safety incidents in England. Resuscitation 2014;85(12):1759–63.
41. Dabney BW, Kalisch BJ. Nurse staffing levels and patient-reported missed nursing care. J Nurs Care Qual 2015;30(4):306–12.
42. Needleman J, Buerhaus P, Mattke S, et al. Nurse-staffing levels and the quality of care in hospitals. N Engl J Med 2002;346(22):1715–22.

43. Aiken LH, Clarke SP, Sloane DM, et al. Effects of hospital care environment on patient mortality and nurse outcomes. J Nurs Adm 2008;38(5):223–9.
44. National Institute of Nursing Research. Changing practice, changing lives: 10 landmark nursing research studies. Available at: https://www.ninr.nih.gov/sites/www.ninr.nih.gov/files/10-landmark-nursing-research-studies.pdf. Accessed March 30, 2016.
45. Hamilton P, Eschiti VS, Hernandez K, et al. Differences between weekend and weekday nurse work environments and patient outcomes: a focus group approach to model testing. J Perinat Neonatal Nurs 2007;21(4):331–41.
46. Teclaw R, Osatuke K. Nurse perceptions of workplace environment: differences across shifts. J Nurs Manag 2015;23(8):1137–46.
47. Smith KK, Gilcreast D, Pierce K. Evaluation of staff's retention of ACLS and BLS skills. Resuscitation 2008;78:59–65.
48. Shearer B, Marshall S, Buist MD, et al. What stops hospital clinical staff from following protocols? An analysis of the incidence and factors behind the failure of bedside clinical staff to activate the rapid response system in a multi-campus Australian metropolitan healthcare service. BMJ Qual Saf 2012;21(7):569–75.
49. Izadnegahdar M, Mackay M, Lee MK, et al. Sex and ethnic differences in outcomes of acute coronary syndrome and stable angina patients with obstructive coronary artery disease. Circ Cardiovasc Qual Outcomes 2016;9(1):S26–35.
50. Mian Z, Wei J, Bharadwaj M, et al. Prior myocardial infarction is associated with coronary endothelial dysfunction in women with signs and symptoms of ischemia and no obstructive coronary artery disease. Int J Cardiol 2016;207:137–9.

Moving?

Make sure your subscription moves with you!

To notify us of your new address, find your **Clinics Account Number** (located on your mailing label above your name), and contact customer service at:

Email: journalscustomerservice-usa@elsevier.com

800-654-2452 (subscribers in the U.S. & Canada)
314-447-8871 (subscribers outside of the U.S. & Canada)

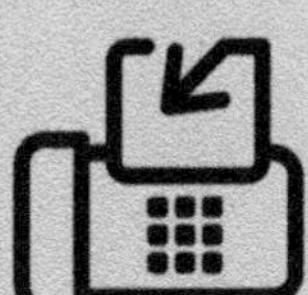

Fax number: 314-447-8029

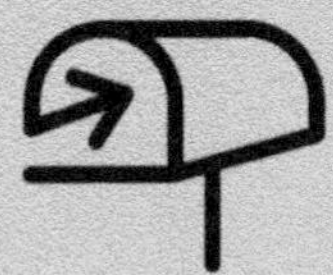

Elsevier Health Sciences Division
Subscription Customer Service
3251 Riverport Lane
Maryland Heights, MO 63043

*To ensure uninterrupted delivery of your subscription, please notify us at least 4 weeks in advance of move.

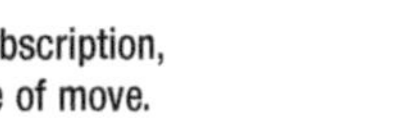

Printed and bound by CPI Group (UK) Ltd, Croydon, CR0 4YY
03/10/2024
01040395-0013